EMERGENCY CARE
Medical and Trauma Scenarios

EMERGENCY CARE
Medical and Trauma Scenarios

Michael David Greenberg, M.D.
Resident in Internal Medicine
New York University Medical Center:
University Hospital
Bellevue Hospital
Veterans Administration Hospital
New York, New York

Joseph J. Lieber, M.D.
Fellow in Nephrology
St. Luke's-Roosevelt Medical Center;
Affiliate
Columbia University College of Physicians and Surgeons
New York, New York

J.B. Lippincott Philadelphia
London   Mexico City   New York
St. Louis   São Paulo   Sydney

Acquisitions Editor: Patricia L. Cleary
Manuscript Editor: Diana Merritt
Design Coordinator: Caren Erlichman
Designer: Terri Siegel
Cover Design: Kevin Curry
Production Manager: Carol A. Florence
Production Coordinator: Kathryn Rule
Compositor: Digitype, Inc.
Text Printer/Binder: R.R. Donnelly & Sons Company
Cover Printer: Phoenix Color Corp.

Copyright © 1989 by J.B. Lippincott Company.

All rights reserved. No part of this book may be used or reproduced in any manner whatsoever without permission except for brief quotations embodied in critical articles and reviews. Printed in the United States of America. For information write J.B. Lippincott Company, East Washington Square, Philadelphia, Pennsylvania 19105.

6 5 4 3 2 1

Library of Congress Cataloging-in-Publication Data

Greenberg, Michael David.
    Emergency care : medical and trauma scenarios / Michael David Greenberg, Joseph J. Lieber.
       p. cm.
    Includes bibliographies.
    ISBN 0-397-54624-6
    1. Medical emergencies—Problems, exercises, etc.   2. Medical emergencies—Case studies.   I. Title.
    [DNLM: 1. Allied Health Personnel.   2. Emergencies—problems.   3. Emergency Medical Services—problems.   4. First Aid—problems. WX 18 G798e]
RC86.9.G74 1989
610.73′61—dc19
DNLM/DLC
for Library of Congress   88-13947
                                                                                            CIP

The authors and publisher have exerted every effort to ensure that drug selection and dosage set forth in this text are in accord with current recommendations and practice at the time of publication. However, in view of ongoing research, changes in government regulations, and the constant flow of information relating to drug therapy and drug reactions, the reader is urged to check the package insert for each drug for any change in indications and dosage and for added warnings and precautions. This is particularly important when the recommended agent is a new or infrequently employed drug.

    Any procedure or practice described in this book should be applied by the health-care practitioner under appropriate supervision in accordance with professional standards of care used with regard to the unique circumstances that apply in each practice situation. Care has been taken to confirm the accuracy of information presented and to describe generally accepted practices. However, the authors, editors and publisher cannot accept any responsibility for errors or omissions or for consequences from application of the information in this book and make no warranty, express or implied, with respect to the contents of the book.

To my wife Mary Theresa, who has always been there for me and whose love and friendship make each day beautiful and my life complete

and

To my loving parents, the greatest mother and father a son could ask for.

Michael David Greenberg

To my loving wife Robin, my daughter Heather and my parents. They have given so generously of their time during the production of this book.

Joseph J. Lieber

Preface

Prehospital emergency medicine has made great strides since its beginnings. Spurred by studies in the early and mid-1960s that demonstrated the need for improved prehospital care, and aided by governmental funding, state and local organizations worked diligently to establish guidelines and training programs to improve prehospital emergency care. Through continued funding, research, and implementation these primitive beginnings have blossomed into an integrated, coherent, and unified entity—the Emergency Medical Services (EMS) system. The level of sophistication of today's EMS system is easily taken for granted until one realizes that it was in the not-too-distant past that "state of the art" prehospital care consisted of little more than rapid transport and words of comfort.

Over the past two decades, prehospital care has reached an increasingly impressive level of sophistication. The number and types of emergency situations that are handled by emergency care personnel have increased dramatically, as have the tools, techniques, and procedures performed outside the hospital "in the field." Today's prehospital health care provider is expected to have not only the wisdom to distinguish the subtle signs of a pulmonary embolism, but also the manual dexterity to "drop a line" or "code a patient," often under the most adverse conditions.

Emergency Care: Medical and Trauma Scenarios is designed both for emergency care personnel in training and for seasoned veterans. We have provided a series of true-to-life case scenarios covering all the basic areas of prehospital emergency medicine. Each scenario will challenge the emergency medical technician to integrate his or her fund of knowledge with clinical acumen.

In each chapter, a short case presentation is followed by a series of clinically related questions. A full discussion of the salient features of the case follows, along with correct answers to the questions. For those who desire to pursue aspects of the case in more detail, we have provided several source references for each question, in the answer section. In most cases, the first cited source provides basic information about the topic, and subsequent references discuss the topic at a more advanced level. Finally, we have provided a short "follow-up" on what happened to the particular patient following admission to the hospital. This format provides the paramedic with a complete overview of how patients' problems are managed, not only in the ambulance but also once they arrive at the hospital.

In selecting the case scenarios and associated materials, we have made every effort to cover the most pertinent areas of prehospital emergency medicine in accordance with the new, revised Department of Transportation National Standard Paramedic Training Curricula and the recent American Heart Association Advanced Cardiac Life Support (ACLS) training protocols. We hope that *Emergency Care* will provide a rich source of materials for students, emergency care personnel, and instructors alike.

Michael David Greenberg, M.D.
Joseph J. Lieber, M.D.

Acknowledgments

We would like to acknowledge the many hours of hard work spent by our friends, families, and colleagues in helping to bring this work to fruition.

To Patricia Cleary, our editor at J.B. Lippincott, we are extremely grateful. Her enthusiasm, patience, and expertise have been of immeasurable value in the development and preparation of this work. To Diana Merritt we also extend our deepest appreciation for her meticulous work as manuscript editor.

A special thanks is in order to William Morse, Paul Maguire, Charlie Howe and Robert Madigan of Mary Immaculate Hospital in New York City for their never ending support and encouragement. To the paramedics and EMTs of 42G, 42F, and 42W we extend our deepest appreciation. Their dedication, professionalism, and talent have been both educational and inspirational.

The technical preparation of this manuscript would have been impossible without the help of Robert A. Greenberg and Mary Theresa Greenberg, who spent many a sleepless night and countless hours typing, numbering, proofing, and collating.

We kindly thank the staff of *The Journal of Emergency Care and Transportation* for allowing us permission to draw upon works previously published by the authors in their periodical. Specifically, Chapters 7, 9, 11, 12, 13, 14, and 26 have been modified from materials published in a monthly column written by the authors.

We are grateful to Jane Huff, David P. Doernbach, and Roger D. White, authors of *ECG Workout: Exercises in Arrhythmia Interpretation*, for graciously allowing us to reproduce many of the EKG tracings in their text.

Finally, we owe the greatest thanks to our wives Mary Theresa (M.D.G.) and Robin (J.J.L.) for standing by our sides throughout the preparation of this work and giving so generously of their time. Their love, encouragement, and support made this work possible.

Contents

MEDICAL EMERGENCIES

1. Chest Pain in an Elderly Man 3
2. A 78-Year-Old Man with Dyspnea 17
3. Altered Mental State and Fever in a College Student 25
4. Dyspnea and Rash in a Young Woman 37
5. A Syncopal Episode in a Chronic Alcoholic 49
6. Chest Pain and Palpitations in a Middle-Aged Man 61
7. An Unconscious Man with Impending Respiratory Failure 71
8. Cough and Fever in a Young Woman 83
9. Chest Pain and Dyspnea 93

TRAUMA EMERGENCIES

10. Acute Respiratory Distress Following a Stab Wound to the Chest 105
11. Orthopedic Injuries in a Multiple Trauma Victim 111
12. Penetrating Abdominal Trauma in a Young Man 119
13. Thermal Injuries in a 28-Year-Old Man 127
14. Thoracoabdominal Pain Following a Fall 141

ADVANCED CARDIAC LIFE SUPPORT EMERGENCIES

15. Palpitations and Dyspnea 151
16. Hypotension and an Altered Mental State in an Elderly Woman 157
17. Palpitations in a Middle-Aged Man 167
18. Acute Chest Pain Followed by Cardiopulmonary Arrest 173
19. Cardiac Arrest with Multiple Malignant Arrhythmias 181
20. Dizziness in an Elderly Man 187

PEDIATRIC EMERGENCIES

21 Acute Respiratory Distress in an Infant 195
22 Cough and Fever in a Pediatric Patient 199
23 Cardiopulmonary Arrest in a Pediatric Patient 211
24 Upper Extremity Injury in a 5-Year-Old Boy 217
25 A 3-Year-Old Child with Sudden Shortness of Breath 223

OBSTETRIC–GYNECOLOGIC EMERGENCIES

26 Abdominal Pain, Weakness, and Hypotension in a
    Teenage Woman 233

MEDICAL EMERGENCIES

1

Chest Pain in an Elderly Man

You and your partner receive a call to "respond for" an "elderly male with chest pain." After a 15-minute response interval you pull up in front of a small private house. You are directed into the living room by a middle-aged woman who tells you that her husband has been having terrible chest pain. As you question your patient, your partner begins his physical examination.

Your patient is a mildly obese 58-year-old man weighing approximately 220 pounds. He tells you that he is having severe chest pain, which he describes as a "sharp ache." The pain is generalized over the anterior precordium although he also states that it seems to "go through to his back." He tells you that it began approximately 1 hour ago while he was watching television and that it was associated with nausea and with three episodes of vomiting. The pain has been continuous since its start. Its intensity is not altered by exaggerated breathing, body movements, or rest. Your patient reports that this is the first time he has ever experienced these symptoms.

Medical history reveals hypertension for the past 20 years, occasional migraine headaches, and an appendectomy at age 23. His medications include hydrochlorothiazide 25 mg po bid, propranolol 60 mg po bid, clonidine 0.20 mg bid, and acetaminophen 325 mg as needed. Your patient states that he has smoked one and one half packs of cigarettes a day for the past 40 years and that he drinks alcohol moderately. He works as a postal clerk. He reports no medication allergies.

Physical examination reveals an alert individual in moderate distress. Vital signs upon arrival are BP (right arm, sitting) 140/90, pulse 120 regular and weak, respiration 26 regular and shallow, and temperature cool to touch. Head and neck examination shows pupils to be equal, round, and reactive to light. Conjunctiva are pale and sclera are nonicteric. His neck is supple and has no palpable masses, and the trachea is midline. The thorax is normal in size and contour and there is symmetrical respiratory excursion. No signs of external trauma are observable and there is no pain upon palpation of the precordium.

Auscultation reveals bilaterally normal breath sounds in both anterior and posterior lung fields. No adventitial sounds are heard and a pleural friction rub is absent. Cardiac examination shows the point of maximal intensity (PMI) to be normally placed. Heart sounds are normal S_1S_2 although somewhat diminished in intensity. No gallops or murmurs are auscultated and a pericardial friction rub is absent. Jugular venous distension (JVD) is absent with the patient in a sitting position, and hepatojugular reflux (HJR) is absent. The abdominal examination is

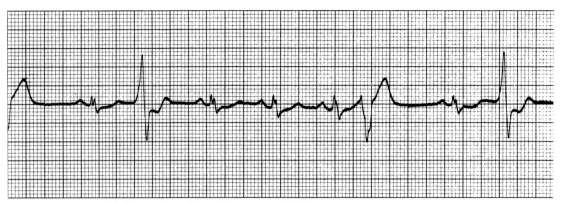

FIGURE 1-1. Lead II EKG recorded shortly after arrival at the scene.

unremarkable although a scar is noted in the patient's lower right abdominal quadrant. His extremities show no signs of edema although peripheral cyanosis and poor capillary refill of the fingernail beds are seen. Your patient's skin is cool to touch and he is markedly diaphoretic. Gross neurologic examination reveals an alert and oriented, although somewhat anxious, individual. No focal neurologic findings are noted.

Vital signs repeated 8 minutes after your arrival are BP (right arm, sitting) 134/86, pulse 128 regular and shallow, respiration 24 regular and shallow, and temperature cool to touch. Cardiac monitoring is begun and a rhythm strip is recorded (Figure 1-1). Medical control is contacted and appropriate treatment is instituted. Following treatment, your patient's EKG rhythm is that depicted in Figure 1-2. Transport to the nearest hospital follows with an estimated arrival time 20 minutes later.

When you and your patient arrive at the emergency room, his blood is drawn for chemical analysis, a full 12 lead cardiogram is ordered, and blood is sent for cardiac enzyme measurement.

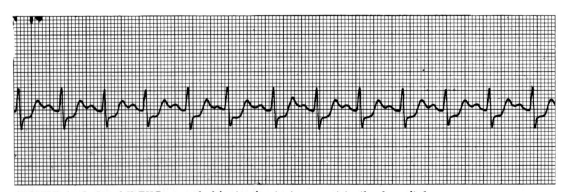

FIGURE 1-2. Lead II EKG recorded just prior to transport to the hospital.

Questions

Read each question carefully, keeping in mind the context of the case under discussion. Select the best answer from the choices presented.

1. Which of the following is best documented as your patient's chief complaint?
   A. Nausea
   B. Headache
   C. Chest pain
   D. Hypertension
   E. Back pain

2. In a patient complaining of chest pain it is important to determine all of the following except
   A. Intensity (mild, moderate, severe)
   B. Associated manifestations (headache, nausea, blurred vision)
   C. Aggravating and relieving factors (breathing, rest, nitroglycerin)
   D. Presence of blurred vision
   E. Chronology (duration, constancy, chronicity)
   F. Setting in which the pain occurred (at rest, during physical exercise, while having an argument)
   G. Quality of the pain (crushing, burning, aching)

3. Which of the following questions would be least effective in your initial attempts to establish the characteristics of your patient's chest pain?
   A. "What were you doing when the pain started?"
   B. "Does anything you do seem to make the pain feel better?"
   C. "Could you describe to me what the pain feels like?"
   D. "Does the pain radiate to your left shoulder and arm?"
   E. "Where exactly do you feel the pain?"

4. Which of the following statements incorrectly pairs one of your patient's medications with either its trade name or its dominant pharmaceutical action?
   A. Hydrochlorothiazide—Lasix—a diuretic
   B. Propranolol—Inderal—a β-adrenergic blocker
   C. Clonidine—Catapres—an antihypertensive
   D. Acetaminophen—Tylenol—an analgesic

5. Which of the following correctly describes the flow of blood from the systemic venous system to the systemic arterial system?
   A. Superior and inferior vena cava, right atrium, mitral valve, right ventricle, pulmonic valve, pulmonary artery, lungs, pulmonary vein, left atrium, tricuspid valve, left ventricle, aortic valve, aorta
   B. Superior and inferior vena cava, right atrium, tricuspid valve, right ventricle, pulmonic valve, pulmonary vein, lungs, pulmonary artery, left atrium, mitral valve, left ventricle, aortic value, aorta

C. Superior and inferior vena cava, right atrium, pulmonic valve, right ventricle, tricuspid valve, pulmonary artery, lungs, pulmonary vein, left atrium, mitral valve, left ventricle, aortic valve, aorta
D. Superior and inferior vena cava, right atrium, tricuspid valve, right ventricle, pulmonic valve, pulmonary artery, lungs, pulmonary vein, left atrium, mitral valve, left ventricle, aortic valve, aorta
E. Superior and inferior vena cava, right atrium, tricuspid valve, right ventricle, pulmonic valve, pulmonary artery, lungs, coronary arteries, left atrium, mitral valve, left ventricle, aortic valve, aorta

6. Your patient's initial blood pressure reading of 140/90 reflects which of the following?
   A. Systolic arterial pressure = 140 mm Hg, diastolic arterial pressure = 90 mm Hg, pulse pressure = 50 mm Hg, mean arterial pressure = 107 mm Hg
   B. Systolic arterial pressure = 140 mm Hg, diastolic arterial pressure = 90 mm Hg, pulse pressure = 230 mm Hg, mean arterial pressure = 107 mm Hg
   C. Systolic venous pressure = 140 mm Hg, diastolic venous pressure = 90 mm Hg, pulse pressure = 50 mm Hg, mean venous pressure = 107 mm Hg
   D. Systolic arterial pressure = 90 mm Hg, diastolic arterial pressure = 140 mm Hg, pulse pressure = 115 mm Hg, mean arterial pressure = 107 mm Hg

7. The removal of waste products and the provision of oxygen and other nutrients to the heart muscle is accomplished primarily through the
   A. Coronary arteries
   B. Pulmonary arteries
   C. Blood in the right atrium
   D. Blood in the left ventricle
   E. Temporal artery

8. Risk factors exhibited by your patient that are associated with the development of cardiovascular disease include all of the following except
   A. Hypertension
   B. Cigarette smoking
   C. Moderate use of alcohol
   D. Family history of cardiovascular disease

9. Chest pain is frequently encountered as the chief complaint with each of the following conditions except
   A. Dissecting aortic aneurysm
   B. Angina pectoris
   C. Cor pulmonale
   D. Uncomplicated acute myocardial infarction

10. The chest pain of myocardial infarction is characterized by all of the following except
    A. Failure to be relieved by rest

B. Moderate to severe intensity
   C. Duration of less then ten minutes
   D. Frequent occurrence while at rest
   E. Failure to be easily relieved by nitroglycerin

11. Chest pain that comes on with exertion, is relieved by rest and sublingual nitroglycerin, and lasts from 2 to 10 minutes, is most characteristic of
    A. Angina pectoris
    B. Pulmonary embolism
    C. Acute myocardial infarction
    D. Dissecting aortic aneurysm
    E. Pneumonia

12. Which of the following formed blood elements has as its predominant function the transport of oxygen?
    A. Erythrocyte
    B. Thrombocyte
    C. Granular leukocyte (neutrophil)
    D. Lymphocyte

13. Your patient's clinical condition is most consistent with which of the following presumptive field diagnoses?
    A. Acute pulmonary edema
    B. Angina pectoris
    C. Acute myocardial infarction
    D. Congestive heart failure
    E. Dissecting aortic aneurysm

14. In a patient complaining of chest pain the most useful information in arriving at a correct field diagnosis is
    A. The patient's vital signs
    B. A detailed physical examination
    C. The patient's electrocardiogram
    D. A good medical history

15. The most common cause of early death in a patient who has suffered a myocardial infarction is
    A. Cardiogenic shock
    B. Acute pulmonary edema
    C. Cardiac arrhythmias
    D. Rupture of the ventricular myocardium

16. Medically sound treatment of your patient may include each of the following except
    A. Frequent monitoring of vital signs
    B. Establishment of an intravenous line

C. Administration of oxygen
D. Administration of an appropriate anti-arrhythmic agent
E. Constant cardiac monitoring
F. Intravenous administration of a diuretic

17. Your patient's initial cardiac rhythm (Figure 1-1) is best classified as
    A. Underlying sinus rhythm with premature atrial beats
    B. Normal sinus rhythm with aberrant conduction
    C. Second degree AV heart block with premature ventricular beats
    D. Underlying sinus rhythm with bundle branch block and multifocal premature ventricular beats

18. Management of your patient's initial cardiac rhythm (Figure 1-1) is best implemented by
    A. No medication necessary; supportive measures and monitoring only
    B. Establishment of a dopamine infusion at 2 to 5 ug/kg/min
    C. Administration of lidocaine as a 75 to 100 mg intravenous bolus followed by a 2 to 4 mg/min drip
    D. Administration of atropine sulfate, 0.5 mg by intravenous bolus repeated at 5-minute intervals up to a maximum of 2 mg
    E. No medication necessary; careful monitoring and carotid sinus massage

19. Following initial treatment, your patient continues to complain of severe chest pain. You contact medical control and discuss the possibility of administering an analgesic medication. Medications frequently used as analgesics in treating chest pain due to suspected acute myocardial infarction include
    A. Naloxone and aspirin
    B. Nitrous oxide and morphine sulfate
    C. Furosemide and atropine sulfate
    D. Nitroglycerin and oxygen

20. An EKG rhythm strip recorded 5 minutes into transport shows the rhythm depicted in Figure 1-2. This rhythm is best classified as
    A. Junctional tachycardia
    B. Normal sinus rhythm
    C. Sinus tachycardia
    D. Second degree AV heart block

21. Which of the following sets of findings most clearly suggests a toxic reaction to lidocaine?
    A. Drowsiness, numbness, confusion, and seizures
    B. Double vision, tachycardia, numbness, headache
    C. Confusion, incontinence, hallucinations, hypertension
    D. Itching, drowsiness, tachypnea, impaired color vision

22. If your patient should develop dyspnea, bilateral rales, jugular venous disten-

sion (JVD), and an S₃ gallop, a reasonable medication to consider administering would be
   A. Furosemide
   B. Isoproterenol
   C. Atropine
   D. Diazepam

23. Early complications to be watched for following admission of your patient to the hospital include all of the following except
   A. Arrhythmias
   B. Rupture of the ventricular septal wall
   C. Cardiogenic shock
   D. Bacterial endocarditis

24. Myocardial infarction involving damage to which of the following portions of the heart is most likely to be complicated by cardiogenic shock?
   A. Anterior wall
   B. Pure posterior wall
   C. Inferior wall
   D. Subendocardial

25. Measurement of blood levels of which of the following sets of enzymes is helpful in documenting the occurrence of a recent myocardial infarction?
   A. Aldolase, lactate dehydrogenase (LDH), serum glutamic-oxaloacetic transaminase (SGOT)
   B. Creatine phosphokinase (CPK), serum glutamic-oxaloacetic transaminase (SGOT), lactate dehydrogenase (LDH)
   C. Serum glutamic-pyruvic transaminase (SGPT), creatine phosphokinase (CPK), lactate dehydrogenase (LDH)
   D. Amylase, creatine phosphokinase (CPK), lactate dehydrogenase (LDH)

26. Approximately ½ hour after transporting your patient to the emergency room, your partner decides to see how he is doing. After returning from the ER he tells you that the patient seems much better and his "cardiac enzymes came back normal" but that the physician in charge has ordered him kept for further observation. Your partner turns to you and, seeming a little puzzled, asks you, "If his cardiac enzymes are normal, why are they keeping him for observation?" Your best response would be
   A. Measuring cardiac enzymes is of little diagnostic value
   B. There was probably a laboratory error in measuring your patient's cardiac enzymes
   C. Abnormalities in cardiac enzymes are often not apparent if measured in the first hour or so after an acute myocardial infarction, so enzymes must be periodically reevaluated
   D. The administration of high concentration oxygen often masks abnormalities in cardiac enzymes

27. A patient who has sustained a major transmural myocardial infarction would most likely show EKG abnormalities related to all of the following except
   A. P waves
   B. ST segment
   C. T waves
   D. Q waves

Discussion

Acute myocardial infarction (AMI) is an established cause of morbidity and mortality in the Western world and is frequently encountered in most emergency medical services (EMS) systems. Since the principal causes of death in the hours immediately following an AMI are related to the development of arrhythmias (especially malignant ventricular arrhythmias), the ability of prehospital EMS personnel to recognize and treat both myocardial infarctions and related complications is vital.

The term *acute myocardial infarction,* or in layman's terms, a "heart attack," denotes death (necrosis) of cardiac muscle tissue (myocardium) resulting from an imbalance between the supply and demand of oxygen to the heart. Normally, oxygen is carried to the myocardium bound to hemoglobin inside red blood cells (erythrocytes). Blood vessels known as the coronary arteries originate from the aorta and divide into a series of branches, each supplying a given portion of the heart tissue. When a blockage occurs in one of these vessels, the blood supply to a portion of the heart is compromised. The result is that oxygen and other nutrients cannot reach the tissue, nor can metabolic waste products be removed from that area of the myocardium. This combination results in various degrees of myocardial injury and necrosis (infarction).

Although atypical presentations are quite common and "silent myocardial infarctions" (myocardial infarctions in the absence of pain) are being recognized with much greater frequency, the classical picture of a myocardial infarction will usually include a chief complaint of squeezing or pressurelike chest pain that is substernal in location and often radiates to the arms, shoulder, or jaw, and is of moderate to severe intensity. Often the pain begins while the patient is at rest and is accompanied by varying degrees of nausea, vomiting, diaphoresis, and extreme anxiety. Because other chest pain syndromes may present with similar symptomatology, a careful physical examination and complete medical history are essential to establish a field diagnosis of AMI (Table 1–1).

In the present case the patient's clinical presentation is consistent with a presumptive field diagnosis of AMI. Other clinical syndromes to be considered include angina pectoris, congestive heart failure (CHF), dissecting aortic aneurysm, and acute pulmonary emboli (APE). The latter normally presents with the combination of pleuritic chest pain (pain that worsens when the patient inspires), tachypnea, and hemoptysis. None of these findings are present in the case at hand. CHF classically presents with signs and symptoms referable to increased pulmonary and systemic congestion. Since jugular venous distension (JVD), hepatojugular reflux

TABLE 1-1. Differential Diagnostic Features of Chest Pain

	Myocardial Infarction	Angina Pectoris	Dissecting Aneurysm	Pericarditis
Quality	Viselike pressure, heaviness, indigestion	Pressure, ache, discomfort, squeezing	Tearing, ripping	Sharp, stabbing
Severity	Moderate to severe	Mild to moderate	Severe	Variable
Location	Retrosternal	Retrosternal	Anterior chest	Retrosternal
Radiation	Left or right arm, shoulders, jaw, neck, oropharynx	Left or right arm, shoulders, jaw, neck, oropharynx	Back	Left or right arm, shoulders, jaw, neck
Chronology	Sudden onset, prolonged duration (often greater than 15 min)	Sudden onset, short duration (often less than 3 min)	Sudden onset, lasts for hours	Sudden onset, lasts for several days
Precipitating Factors	Onset at rest or during sleep is common	Exertion, stress, cold, large food intake	Hypertension	Recent infection, uremia, heart surgery, myocardial infarction
Aggravating Factors		Exertion		Deep breathing, coughing, supine position
Relieving Factors	Opiate analgesics	Nitroglycerin, rest	Large doses of opiate analgesics	Upright and bent forward posture
Associated Manifestations	Nausea, vomiting, dyspnea, sense of "impending doom," S_4, EKG changes	S_3, paradoxical split of S_2, dyspnea, EKG changes with ST segment depression or elevation	Pulsus paradoxus, asymmetrical blood pressure readings	Friction rub, EKG changes

(HJR), pitting peripheral edema, and rales and rhonchi were all absent, the diagnosis of CHF is similarly unlikely. In considering the possibility of angina pectoris it is important to obtain a detailed description of the following aspects of the patient's pain: quality (stabbing, pulsating, pressurelike), quantity (mild, moderate, or severe intensity), location, radiation, chronology (constancy and duration), aggravating and relieving factors (rest, nitroglycerin, cold, breathing), and any associated manifestations (nausea, vomiting, shortness of breath). The pain of angina pectoris is characteristically brought on by exertion, relieved by rest and nitroglycerin, and of short duration.

In the case at hand the pain is reported to have begun while the patient was at rest, did not abate with cessation of activity, and is of long duration. These findings do not suggest an attack of angina pectoris, but are more characteristic of the pain accompanying myocardial infarction. Because pain which radiates to the back between the scapulae accompanies dissecting aortic aneurysm, this possibility must also be considered. This pain, however, is classically described as having a "tearing or ripping" quality unlike the "sharp ache" described by the patient. Further arguing against the diagnosis of dissecting aortic aneurysm is the lack of significant vascular findings, such as unequal or diminished pulses, differing blood pressure readings on the right and left arms, or a pulsating abdominal mass. In summary, the patient's clinical symptomatology in conjunction with his multiple risk factors — hypertension, cigarette use, and a family history — make the field diagnosis of AMI a strong one.

Management of this patient and others with suspected myocardial infarction is aimed at preventing further myocardial injury, maintaining an adequate hemodynamic status, and correcting any secondary complications, such as arrhythmias, cardiogenic shock, and CHF. Vital signs should be measured and recorded at frequent intervals. Administer oxygen as soon as possible, using either a face mask or nasal cannula, with the flow rate determined by the severity of the patient's clinical condition. Consider whether the patient has a history of underlying chronic obstructive pulmonary disease (COPD).

Cardiac monitoring using a portable EKG is advisable; record an initial rhythm strip for evaluation and comparison with strips recorded later at the hospital. Establish an intravenous (IV) line with D5/W at a keep-vein-open (KVO) rate to assure easy administration of either medications or fluids should such be necessary. Because the pain and anxiety experienced by many myocardial infarction patients may place an increased burden on an already injured heart, proper reassurance of the patient and use of appropriate pain medication are called for. Depending upon training, local protocols, and the patient's clinical condition, analgesic medications used in cases of suspected myocardial infarction include nitroglycerin, nitrous oxide, morphine sulfate, and varying combinations of these agents.

Examination of your patient's cardiac rhythm (Figure 1-1) reveals an underlying sinus rhythm with frequent multifocal premature ventricular contractions. Since the presence of premature ventricular contractions in the case of suspected AMI is believed by many to be a forewarning of possibly lethal ventricular arrhythmias, such as ventricular fibrillation and ventricular tachycardia, treatment with an appropriate anti-arrhythmic medication is called for. Currently, the drug of choice for field treatment of premature ventricular contractions is lidocaine. Lidocaine is an anti-arrhythmic medication used primarily in treating ventricular arrhythmias, especially those arising in cases of myocardial infarction or digitalis intoxication. Lidocaine inhibits ventricular ectopy (abnormal impulse formation) and reentry (abnormal impulse conduction), the two major causes of malignant ventricular arrhythmias such as ventricular premature contractions, ventricular fibrillation, and ventricular tachycardia. Since lidocaine has little effect upon the SA node, atrial tissue, or AV node, its usefulness is restricted primarily to treating arrhythmias arising within the ventricles.

Because lidocaine is broken down in the liver, any condition which either adversely affects liver function (cirrhosis) or impairs blood flow to the liver (CHF) will slow the rate at which the drug is removed from the body. Failure to consider this fact when determining the dose of lidocaine may lead to administering doses that cause toxic levels of the medication to accumulate. For this reason, the use of lidocaine to treat patients with cirrhosis or CHF, although not contraindicated, must be undertaken with caution, and dosages must be adjusted appropriately.

Whenever lidocaine is used, it is important to recognize and to watch for signs and symptoms of a toxic reaction. These symptoms are primarily referable to the central nervous system and include drowsiness, confusion, numbness, and tingling. In cases of severe toxic reaction, seizures, coma, and cardiac as well as respiratory depression may occur.

The use of lidocaine in the field calls for IV administration in the form of a bolus (rapid administration of a large amount of medication), followed immediately by a continuous lidocaine infusion. Because lidocaine is rapidly inactivated by the body, the initial medication administered as a bolus will have a therapeutic effect limited to between 10 and 20 minutes. In order to maintain the plasma concentration of lidocaine at a steady and therapeutically effective level it is necessary to follow the bolus with a continuous infusion. As the initial bolus medication is inactivated, the medication from the infusion takes over. Therapeutic plasma levels of lidocaine range from approximately 1.5 to 5 ug/ml. Several dosage regimens have been designed to rapidly establish and then maintain this level. A regimen described in many standard texts calls for an initial bolus of 50 to 100 mg (1 mg/kg) followed by a continuous lidocaine infusion at 1 to 4 mg/min (15–50 ug/kg/min) for an average adult weighing 70 kg.

> **Field Diagnosis**
> - Acute myocardial infarction
>
> **Hospital Diagnosis**
> - Extensive anterior wall myocardial infarction

Patient Follow-Up

The patient was admitted to the coronary care unit (CCU) for observation, with the diagnosis of an extensive anterior wall myocardial infarction. He experienced several episodes of ventricular tachycardia during the first 48 hours and was maintained on a lidocaine infusion. On the seventh day he was transferred to the floors, where he continued to show steady improvement. Two weeks after admission to the hospital he was discharged with instructions to return for follow-up.

Answers

1. C
   Caroline NL: Emergency Care in the Streets, 3rd ed, pp 39–42. Boston, Little, Brown & Co, 1987

2. D
   Caroline NL: Emergency Care in the Streets, 3rd ed, pp 40–42. Boston, Little, Brown & Co, 1987

3. **D**

Bates B: A Guide to Physical Examination, 4th ed, p 14. Philadelphia, JB Lippincott, 1987

Greenberg MD: Assessing patient history. J Emerg Serv 14(11):26–28, 1982

4. **A**

Caroline NL: Emergency Care in the Streets, 3rd ed, pp 130–158. Boston, Little, Brown & Co, 1987

5. **D**

Caroline NL: Emergency Care in the Streets, 3rd ed, pp 252–258. Boston, Little, Brown & Co, 1987

Huszar RJ: Emergency Cardiac Care, pp 12–14. Bowie, MD, Robert J Brady Co, 1974

6. **A**

Huszar RJ: Emergency Cardiac Care, p 57. Bowie, MD, Robert J Brady Co, 1974

Guyton AC: Textbook of Medical Physiology, 6th ed, p 221. Philadelphia, WB Saunders, 1981

7. **A**

Caroline NL: Emergency Care in the Streets, 3rd ed, pp 252–262. Boston, Little, Brown & Co, 1987

Huszar RJ: Emergency Cardiac Care, p 13. Bowie, MD, Robert J Brady Co, 1974

8. **C**

Caroline NL: Emergency Care in the Streets, 3rd ed, pp 264–74. Boston, Little, Brown & Co, 1987

American Heart Association: Standards and guidelines for cardiopulmonary resuscitation (CPR) and emergency cardiac care (ECC). JAMA 255:2905, 1986

9. **C**

Gore JM, Dalen JE: Cor pulmonale. Hosp Med 19:39, 1983

Andreoli TE, Carpenter CCJ, Plum F (eds): Essentials of Medicine, pp 11–12. Philadelphia, WB Saunders, 1986

10. **C**

Caroline NL: Emergency Care in the Streets, 3rd ed, pp 252–72. Boston, Little, Brown & Co, 1987

Andreoli TE, Carpenter CCJ, Plum F (eds): Cecil's Essentials of Medicine, pp 10–12. Philadelphia, WB Saunders, 1986

11. **A**

Caroline NL: Emergency Care in the Streets, 3rd ed, pp 258–72. Boston, Little, Brown & Co, 1987

Willerson JT: Angina pectoris. In Wyngaarden JB, Smith LH Jr (eds): Textbook of Medicine, 18th ed, pp 323–329. Philadelphia, WB Saunders, 1988

12. **A**

Caroline NL: Emergency Care in the Streets, 3rd ed, pp 30–31. Boston, Little, Brown & Co, 1987

Grant HD, Murray RH Jr, Bergeron JD: Emergency Care, 3rd ed, pp 130–131. Bowie, MD, Robert J Brady Co, 1982

13. **C**

Caroline NL: Emergency Care in the Streets, 3rd ed, pp 264–72. Boston, Little, Brown & Co, 1987

Willerson JT: Acute myocardial infarction. In Wyngaarden JB, Smith LH Jr (eds): Textbook of Medicine, 18th ed, pp 329–337. Philadelphia, WB Saunders, 1985

14. **D**

Andreoli TE, Carpenter CCJ, Plum F (eds): Cecil's Essentials of Medicine, p 10. Philadelphia, WB Saunders, 1986

Greenberg MD: Evaluating the cardiac patient—II. J Emerg Serv 15:18, 1983

15. **C**

Caroline NL: Emergency Care in the Streets, 3rd ed, pp 266–67. Boston, Little, Brown & Co, 1987

American Heart Association: Standards and guidelines for cardiopulmonary resuscitation (CPR) and emergency cardiac care (ECC). JAMA 255:2905, 1986

16. **F**

Caroline NL: Emergency Care in the Streets, 3rd ed, pp 264–74. Boston, Little, Brown & Co, 1987

17. **D**

Huff J, Doernbach DP, White RD: ECG Workout: Exercises in Arrhythmia Interpretation, pp 134, 240 (strip 4.49). Philadelphia, JB Lippincott, 1985

Caroline NL: Emergency Care in the Streets, 3rd ed, pp 283–306. Boston, Little, Brown & Co, 1987

18. **C**

American Heart Association: Standards and guidelines for cardiopulmonary resuscitation (CPR) and emergency cardiac care (ECC). JAMA 255:2905, 1986

19. **B**

Caroline NL: Emergency Care in the Streets, 3rd ed, pp 269–270. Boston, Little, Brown & Co, 1987

20. **C**

Huff J, Doernbach DP, White RD: ECG Workout: Exercises in Arrhythmia Interpretation, pp 26, 216 (strip 1.63). Philadelphia, JB Lippincott, 1985

21. **A**

Caroline NL: Emergency Care in the Streets, 3rd ed, p 145. Boston, Little, Brown & Co, 1987

Miller K: Lidocaine. J Emerg Serv 18:14, 1986

22. **A**

Caroline NL: Emergency Care in the Streets, 3rd ed, pp 264–276. Boston, Little, Brown & Co, 1987

23. **D**

Willerson JT: Acute myocardial infarction. In Wyngaarden JB, Smith LH Jr (eds): Textbook of Medicine, 17th ed, pp 291–293. Philadelphia, WB Saunders, 1985

24. **A**

Willerson JT: Acute myocardial infarction. In Wyngaarden JB, Smith LH Jr (eds): Textbook of Medicine, 17th ed, pp 291–293. Philadelphia, WB Saunders, 1985

25. **B**

Willerson JT: Acute myocardial infarction. In Wyngaarden JB, Smith LH Jr (eds): Textbook of Medicine, 17th ed. Philadelphia, WB Saunders, 1985

Lamb JI, Carlson VR (eds): Handbook of Cardiovascular Nursing, pp 127–128. Philadelphia, JB Lippincott, 1986

26. **C**

Hurst JW, King SB III, Walter PF et al: Atherosclerotic coronary heart disease: Angina pectoris, myocardial infarction, and other manifestations of myocardial ischemia. In Hurst JW (ed): The Heart, 5th ed, pp 1049–1051. New York, McGraw-Hill, 1982

Willerson JT: Acute myocardial infarction. In Wyngaarden JB, Smith LH Jr (eds): Textbook of Medicine, 17th ed, p 291. Philadelphia, WB Saunders, 1985

27. **A**

Dubin D: Rapid Interpretation of EKGs, 3rd ed, pp 204–246, 274. Tampa, Cover Publishing Co, 1974

Willerson JT: Acute myocardial infarction. In Wyngaarden JB, Smith LH Jr (eds): Textbook of Medicine, 17th ed, p 290. Philadelphia, WB Saunders, 1985

Selected Reading

Dunn HM, McComb JM, Kinney CD et al: Prophylactic lidocaine in the early phase of suspected myocardial infarction. Am Heart J 110:353, 1985

Hancock WE: Ischemic heart disease: Acute myocardial infarction. In Federman DD, Rubenstein E (eds): Medicine, Vol I:X, pp 1–22. New York, Scientific American, 1986

Sebaldt RJ, Nattel S, Kreeft JH et al: Lidocaine therapy with an exponentially declining infusion: Clinical evaluation of an optimized dosing technique. Ann Intern Med 101:632, 1984

Willerson JT: Acute myocardial infarction. In Wyngaarden JB, Smith LH Jr (eds): Textbook of Medicine, 17th ed. Philadelphia, WB Saunders, 1985

2

A 78-Year-Old Man with Dyspnea

Your ambulance is dispatched to assist a male with "difficulty breathing." Upon arrival, you find a thin, elderly man seated erect, breathing with pursed lips and appearing in moderate respiratory distress. He relates that although he is usually short of breath owing to his emphysema, he has been having an unusually bad episode of shortness of breath for the past 2 hours. His normal inhaler has provided some relief, but far less than the relief to which he is accustomed. Upon further questioning the patient denies any chest pain or sweating, though he does admit that a brief episode of palpitations occurred at about the time he first experienced difficulty breathing.

Vital signs upon arrival are BP (right arm, supine) 150/94, pulse 110 regular and strong, respiration 20 and regular, and temperature normal to touch. Pupils are equal, 5 mm in diameter, round, and reactive to light.

Your patient denies any past medical history or surgical conditions except for long-standing emphysema, for which he has been hospitalized several times over the past 10 years. No intubation has ever been necessary. His medications include theophylline (Theo-Dur) 300 mg po tid, terbutaline 5 mg po tid, prednisone 5 mg po od, metaproterenol inhaler 2 puffs qid, and beclomethasone inhaler 2 puffs qid. He also receives low concentration supplemental home oxygen therapy. The patient admits he has smoked up to three packs of cigarettes a day for the past 50 years, but denies he smokes today. He denies having any allergies or using alcohol.

Physical examination shows a 78-year-old man weighing approximately 150 pounds who appears anxious and short of breath. Nasal flaring and use of accessory muscles to aid breathing are noted. The mouth and nail beds appear cyanotic. Positive findings include jugular venous distention (JVD) at 90 degrees, 2 plus pitting pedal edema, and an increased thoracic diameter. Heart sounds are normal S_1S_2, although distant. Also noted is a palpable abdominal mass in the upper right quadrant and a positive hepatojugular reflux (HJR). Percussion of the posterior thorax yields hyperresonance over both lung fields, and auscultation reveals a few scattered rhonchi. Clubbing and peripheral cyanosis are absent. Your patient appears alert and oriented to time, place, and person. The remainder of your examination is noncontributory.

Appropriate initial medical treatment is instituted, your patient's cardiac rhythm is monitored (Figure 2–1), and transport begins. Five minutes into transport, your patient starts to complain of palpitations and his skin turns ashen. The cardiac monitor shows the rhythm seen in Figure 2–2. Vital signs at this time are

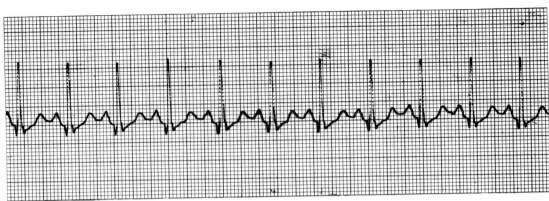

FIGURE 2-1. Lead II EKG recorded upon arrival at the scene.

BP (right arm, sitting) 60 by palpation, radial pulse thready but too fast to count, and respiration 20 and regular. While medical control is contacted, intravenous (IV) fluids are opened to maximum drip rate. A request is made, and permission is granted, to perform an appropriate emergency medical procedure. Upon completion of the procedure, the patient's cardiac rhythm is that shown in Figure 2-3. Accompanying vital signs are BP (left arm, sitting) 110/70, pulse 110 and regular, and respiration 20 and regular. Your patient is now alert and oriented. Transport continues to the hospital without incident and vital signs remain stable.

Questions

Read each question carefully, keeping in mind the context of the case under discussion. Select the best answer from the choices presented.

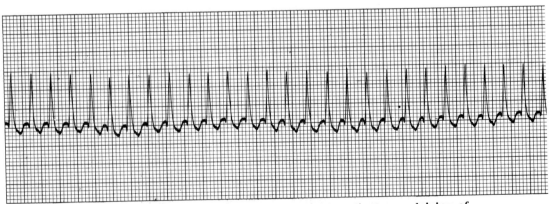

FIGURE 2-2. Lead II EKG recorded during transport with patient complaining of palpitations.

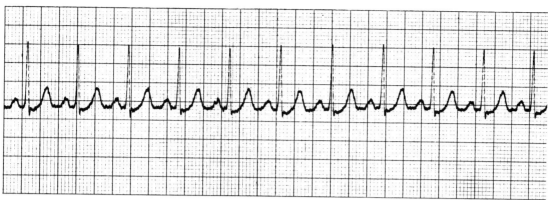

FIGURE 2-3. Lead II EKG recorded following emergency corrective action.

1. The presenting symptom of dyspnea is commonly associated with all of the following except
    A. Delirium tremens
    B. Emphysema
    C. Asthma
    D. Pulmonary edema

2. Indications that your patient is experiencing respiratory distress include all of the following except
    A. Jugular venous distension
    B. Nasal flaring
    C. Pursed lip breathing
    D. Using accessory muscles

3. Clinically, which of the following conditions is best characterized as a reversible episodic bronchospastic disease?
    A. Asthma
    B. Chronic bronchitis
    C. Croup
    D. Emphysema

4. Which of the following is not classified as a chronic obstructive pulmonary disease (COPD)?
    A. Emphysema
    B. Epiglottitis
    C. Asthma
    D. Chronic bronchitis

5. The physical examination findings of jugular venous distension, pedal edema, and positive hepatojugular reflux suggest
    A. Cardiogenic shock

B. Acute myocardial infarction with left ventricular failure
C. Cardiac arrhythmia
D. Cor pulmonale

6. Which of the following pairings incorrectly matches your patient's medication with its pharmacological properties?
    A. Terbutaline—a β-adrenergic agonist
    B. Theo-Dur—a β-adrenergic blocker
    C. Metaproterenol—a β-adrenergic agonist
    D. Prednisone—a systemic glucocorticoid steroid

7. Hyperresonance to percussion in your patient is most likely due to
    A. Increased air trapping in the alveoli
    B. Bilateral pneumothorax
    C. Increased muscle mass of the chest wall
    D. Increased fluid in the alveoli

8. Initial treatment of your patient is best based upon a presumptive field diagnosis of
    A. Acute myocardial infarction with cor pulmonale
    B. Pneumonia
    C. Chronic obstructive pulmonary disease with cor pulmonale
    D. Angina pectoris

9. Basic life support treatment of your patient should include which of the following?
    A. Applying venous constricting bands ("rotating tourniquets")
    B. Increasing inspired CO_2 by having patient rebreathe into a paper bag
    C. Using ammonia inhalants as respiratory stimulants
    D. Administering supplemental oxygen

10. Correct oxygen therapy for your patient is accomplished through
    A. Use of a non-rebreathing face mask with a 10 lpm oxygen supply
    B. Administration of 24% oxygen with a Venturi mask
    C. Use of a nasal cannula with an 8 lpm oxygen supply
    D. Use of Venturi mask set to deliver 60% oxygen
    E. Immediate endotracheal intubation

11. Advanced life support measures should initially include all of the following except
    A. Establishment of a peripheral intravenous line with D5/W
    B. An aminophylline infusion
    C. Cardiac monitoring
    D. Administration of morphine sulfate

12. Your patient's initial EKG (Figure 2-1) is best classified as

A. Normal sinus rhythm
B. Paroxysmal atrial tachycardia
C. Atrial flutter
D. Sinus tachycardia

13. The arrhythmia evidenced by your patient during transport (Figure 2-2) is most correctly called
    A. Sinus tachycardia
    B. Atrial flutter
    C. Atrial fibrillation
    D. Third degree AV block

14. In association with the above arrhythmia (Figure 2-2) you note that your patient's skin is ashen and that his blood pressure has dropped. These changes are most likely the result of
    A. An acute myocardial infarction
    B. Extensive vasoconstriction
    C. A rapid ventricular rate
    D. Increasingly severe hypoxia

15. The procedure approved by medical control is most likely
    A. Nonsynchronized defibrillation at 360 J
    B. Immediate application and inflation of MAST
    C. Synchronized dc cardioversion at 20 J
    D. Use of a 1:10,000 solution of epinephrine, IV bolus

16. Following completion of the procedure referred to in question 15, your patient's cardiac rhythm is that seen in Figure 2-3. This rhythm is
    A. Sinus tachycardia
    B. Multifocal atrial tachycardia
    C. Atrial flutter with a 2:1 AV block
    D. Ventricular tachycardia

Discussion

Your patient's primary symptom is dyspnea. The combination of pursed lip breathing, nasal flaring, and using accessory muscles to aid breathing suggests marked respiratory distress. Shortness of breath, known medically as dyspnea, may be the chief complaint in several medical conditions, including angina pectoris, congestive heart failure (CHF), acute pulmonary edema, pulmonary embolism, and chronic obstructive pulmonary disease (COPD). When a chief complaint of dyspnea is encountered, discovering the cause is greatly aided by carefully questioning the patient about existing medical conditions as well as about medications being taken. In the present case, the patient's report of a substantial smoking history in conjunction with a long-standing history of emphysema strongly suggests that his complaint of shortness of breath is related to an exacerbation of underlying COPD. Although it would be imprudent to attempt a comprehensive discussion of COPD, certain points of clinical relevance are worthy of discussion.

Chronic obstructive pulmonary disease or, as it is sometimes called, chronic obstructive lung disease (COLD), includes chronic bronchitis, emphysema, and according to some specialists, asthma. Emphysema is a pathological condition characterized by enlargement and destruction of the pulmonary acini (respiratory bronchioles, alveolar ducts, and alveolar sacs). Chronic bronchitis is defined in clinical terms by the presence of a chronic cough with sputum production for a minimum of 3 months in at least 2 consecutive years. Asthma is a heterogeneous disorder characterized by episodes of reversible bronchoconstriction. Although the terms "pink puffer" and "blue bloater" are often attached respectively to those with emphysema and chronic bronchitis, their clinical usefulness is limited owing to the wide overlap in symptoms of persons with lung disease.

The findings of jugular venous distention (JVD), hepatojugular reflux (HJR), and pedal edema, in addition to dyspnea, indicate systemic congestion resulting from right-sided heart failure secondary to your patient's underlying pulmonary disease. These cases are known as *cor pulmonale*.

Based on the above discussion, a reasonable field diagnosis for this patient is exacerbation of underlying COPD with cor pulmonale. Treatment of the patient should begin, as always, with ensuring a patent airway and correcting any underlying hypoxia. Oxygen administration is necessary to maintain an adequate blood oxygen level, but must be tempered in view of the history of COPD. Because the respiratory stimulus in many of these patients is a low blood oxygen level ("hypoxic drive") rather than a high carbon dioxide level, administering an enriched oxygen mixture may raise blood oxygen levels to the point where the hypoxic drive is shut off. The results are a decreased respiratory rate, increased hypercapnia, and, in the most extreme cases, respiratory arrest. The goal of oxygen therapy should be to establish a blood oxygen level satisfactory for tissue oxygenation without compromising the patient's hypoxic drive. This result is best achieved by administering a 24% concentration of oxygen, either by using a Venturi mask with the oxygen liter flow set to achieve this concentration or, less precisely but equally effectively, by using a nasal cannula with an oxygen liter flow between 1 and 2 liters/min.

Establishing a peripheral intravenous (IV) line is crucial since these patients frequently require both medication to ease breathing and hydration to compensate for increased loss of fluids. Although the indication and expected response vary considerably from patient to patient, the medication most commonly employed in the field in cases of COPD is aminophylline. This medication is classified as a methylxanthine and probably has multiple actions including bronchodilation and stimulation of the diaphragm. Both these actions lead to an improved ventilatory status. Unfortunately, aminophylline may produce several serious side-effects which must be watched for, including nausea, vomiting, cardiac arrhythmias, and seizures. Other important treatment measures include constant monitoring of vital signs and of the patient's cardiac rhythm. Medications that may either depress respiration or dry out the respiratory tree are best avoided.

The importance of careful cardiac monitoring is exemplified in this case.

Shortly after transport was initiated, your patient underwent sudden hemodynamic deterioration that appears related to the onset of a rapid supraventricular arrhythmia (Figure 2-2). Careful inspection of the rhythm strip shows a rapid, regular rhythm, with no ectopic beats. The narrow QRS complexes imply a supraventricular origin. Although neither P waves nor classic flutter waves are seen, the ventricular rate of 280 to 300 complexes/min indicates that the rhythm is atrial flutter. In most cases of atrial flutter there is a 2:1 or greater conduction ratio, resulting in a slower ventricular response; in the present case, however, it seems that each of the atrial impulses is being conducted through the AV node to the ventricles. The resulting rapid ventricular response is the cause of your patient's sudden hemodynamic deterioration, since the heart is unable to fill sufficiently to maintain an adequate cardiac output. Owing to the potential serious consequences, correcting this rhythm is mandatory. The quickest and most efficacious means for remedying this situation is using low energy dc synchronized cardioversion, which was most probably the procedure recommended by medical control. Following this intervention, the patient becomes hemodynamically stable and clinically improved, and the final EKG reveals a sinus rhythm (Figure 2-3).

Field Diagnosis

- Chronic obstructive pulmonary disease
- Cor pulmonale
- Atrial flutter with 1:1 AV conduction

Hospital Diagnosis

- Chronic obstructive pulmonary disease
- Cor pulmonale

Patient Follow-Up

Because of the complexity of the patient's condition, he was admitted to the intensive care unit (ICU) where his COPD was managed with appropriate medications, including low dose aminophylline, β-adrenergic agonists, intravenous steroids, and nebulizer treatments. His rapid ventricular response to his atrial flutter was attributed to the medications he had been taking. The episode of atrial flutter was attributed to his underlying COPD. Over the next several days he progressed well and was transferred to the regular medical service and discharged 5 days after arriving in the hospital.

Answers

1. A

    Caroline NL: Emergency Care in the Streets, 3rd ed, pp 167-249. Boston, Little, Brown & Co, 1987

2. A

    Caroline NL: Emergency Care in the Streets, 3rd ed, pp 167-249. Boston, Little, Brown & Co, 1987

Cosgriff JH Jr, Ratajczyk C: Respiratory emergencies. In Cosgriff JH Jr, Anderson DL: The Practice of Emergency Care, 2nd ed, pp 210–211. Philadelphia, JB Lippincott, 1984

3. A

Caroline NL: Emergency Care in the Streets, 3rd ed, pp 167–249. Boston, Little, Brown & Co, 1987

Cosgriff JH Jr, Ratajczyk C: Respiratory emergencies. In Cosgriff JH Jr, Anderson DL: The Practice of Emergency Care, 2nd ed, pp 225–227. Philadelphia, JB Lippincott, 1984

4. B

Caroline NL: Emergency Care in the Streets, 3rd ed, pp 167–249. Boston, Little, Brown & Co, 1987

Cosgriff JH Jr, Ratajczyk C: Respiratory emergencies. In Cosgriff JH Jr, Anderson DL: The Practice of Emergency Care, 2nd ed, p 223. Philadelphia, JB Lippincott, 1984

5. D

Gore JM, Dalen JE: Cor pulmonale. Hosp Med 19:39, 1983

Ross JC: Chronic cor pulmonale. In Hurst JW (ed): The Heart, 5th ed, pp 1120–1127. New York, McGraw-Hill, 1982

6. B

Boushey HA, Holtzman MJ: Bronchodilators and other agents used in the treatment of asthma. In Katzung BG (ed): Basic and Clinical Pharmacology, p 208. Los Altos, Lange Medical Publications, 1982

7. A

Caroline NL: Emergency Care in the Streets, 3rd ed, pp 167–249. Boston, Little, Brown & Co, 1987

8. C

Caroline NL: Emergency Care in the Streets, 3rd ed, pp 167–249. Boston, Little, Brown & Co, 1987

Ross JC: Chronic cor pulmonale. In Hurst JW (ed): The Heart, 5th ed, pp 1120–1127. New York, McGraw-Hill, 1982

9. D

Caroline NL: Emergency Care in the Streets, 3rd ed, pp 167–249. Boston, Little, Brown & Co, 1987

10. B

Moser KM: Acute respiratory failure with hypercapnia. In Moser KM, Spragg RG (eds): Respiratory Emergencies, 2nd ed, p 88. St Louis, CV Mosby, 1982

Grant HD, Murray RH Jr, Bergeron JD: Emergency Care, 3rd ed, p 247. Bowie, MD, Robert J Brady Co, 1982

11. D

Caroline NL: Emergency Care in the Streets, 3rd ed, pp 167–249. Boston, Little, Brown & Co, 1987

12. D

Huff J, Doernbach DP, White RD: ECG Workout: Exercises in Arrhythmia Interpretation, pp 14, 214 (strip 1.28). Philadelphia, JB Lippincott, 1985

13. B

Huff J, Doernbach DP, White RD: ECG Workout: Exercises in Arrhythmia Interpretation, pp 43, 219 (strip 2.2). Philadelphia, JB Lippincott, 1985

Alpert MA: Cardiac Arrhythmias, pp 79–92. Chicago, Year Book Medical Publishers, 1980

14. C

Alpert MA: Cardiac Arrhythmias, pp 79–92. Chicago, Year Book Medical Publishers, 1980

15. C

Goldberger E, Wheat MW Jr: Treatment of Cardiac Emergencies, 3rd ed, pp 94–95, 286–293. St Louis, CV Mosby, 1982

16. A

Huff J, Doernbach DP, White RD: ECG Workout: Exercises in Arrhythmia Interpretation, pp 17, 214 (strip 1.36). Philadelphia, JB Lippincott, 1985

Selected Reading

Gore JM, Dalen JE: Cor pulmonale. Hosp Med 19:39, 1983
Hyers TH: Acute respiratory failure. Hosp Med 20:162, 1984

3

Altered Mental State and Fever in a College Student

Your ambulance is dispatched along with the police to aid an emotionally disturbed person. After a 15-minute response interval you arrive and are met by the patient's girlfriend. As you talk with the girlfriend, your partner speaks with the police, who tell him that they were called by a neighbor who saw the patient wandering around in the street. His girlfriend tells you that he was fine last night but that when she came home from work today she found him mumbling and acting bizarre. Further questioning reveals that your patient is an A student at the local college. He does not use any drugs and drinks only socially.

The patient's past medical history includes asthma since childhood, which has been treated with a metaproterenol sulfate (Alupent) inhaler, 2 puffs tid and theophylline (Theo-Dur), 300 mg po bid. He has no allergies and, as far as his girlfriend knows, no psychiatric history.

The patient is a thin, 19-year-old man weighing approximately 175 pounds. He is sitting in the living room mumbling, appears glassy-eyed, and is in no acute distress. Vital signs are BP (right arm, sitting) 100/70, pulse 110 and regular, respiration 18 regular, and temperature warm to touch.

A patent airway is present and there are no signs of foreign matter or secretions in the oropharynx. His trachea is midline and no masses are palpable. Carotid pulses are normal and equal. There is no evidence of splinting and lung sounds are normal and bilaterally clear with good air exchange. Heart sounds are normal S_1S_2 with no extra sounds heard. There is no jugular venous distension (JVD) or peripheral edema. Capillary bed refill is adequate. The abdomen shows no signs of trauma, appears of normal size and shape, and is nondistended. Bowel sounds are slightly hyperactive. The abdomen is soft and nontender. There is no guarding, rebound tenderness, or masses. Extremities are without signs of trauma and show symmetrical and equal pulses. The skin shows no signs of cyanosis or rash.

Your neurologic assessment shows a lethargic individual who is disoriented to time, place, and self. Pupils are round, equal, and reactive to light. Careful observation shows that the eyes do not appear to move in unison. His speech is incoherent. Movement and sensation in all extremities are difficult to assess due to lack of cooperation, but appear grossly normal. Deep tendon reflexes (DTRs) are symmetrically equal. Plantar reflexes show bilateral flexion. Upon flexion of the neck

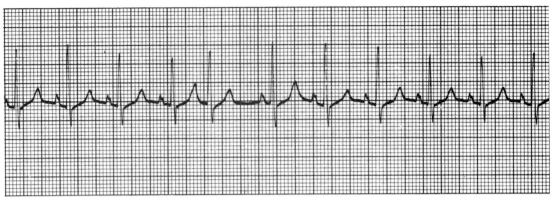

FIGURE 3-1. Lead II EKG recorded shortly after arrival at the scene.

moderate rigidity is noted and the patient complains of pain. No otorrhea, rhinorrhea, Battle's sign, or raccoon's eyes are noted.

Your patient's vital signs are monitored, initial treatment is begun, and his cardiac rhythm is recorded (Figure 3-1). Transportation to the hospital is undertaken with an estimated arrival time 20 minutes later.

Upon arrival to the emergency room the patient is examined by the emergency room medical team. A diagnostic procedure is performed (Table 3-1), blood is drawn for chemical analysis, and a 12 lead cardiogram and chest x-ray are ordered.

Questions

Read each question carefully, keeping in mind the context of the case under discussion. Select the best answer from the choices presented.

1. The maintenance of a constant internal environment by the cells and tissues of the body is called
    A. Homeostasis
    B. Metabolism
    C. Hemostasis
    D. Metastasis

TABLE 3-1. Results of Cerebrospinal Fluid Analysis

Test	Result	Normal Range
Appearance	Cloudy	Clear
Cell Count	1200 WBC/mm^3	0-10 WBC/mm^3
	75% PMNs and 25% mononuclear cells	All mononuclear cells
Glucose	40 mg/dl	45-80 mg/dl
Protein	150 mg/dl	15-45 mg/dl
Bacteria	Numerous	None

2. Basic functions of all mammalian cells include all of the following except
   A. Secretion
   B. Respiration
   C. Conductivity
   D. Margination

3. Which of the following choices correctly lists the different layers of the meninges, starting with the layer directly overlying the brain tissue and working outwards:
   A. Dura mater, arachnoid membrane, pia mater
   B. Arachnoid membrane, dura mater, pia mater
   C. Pia mater, dura mater, arachnoid membrane
   D. Dura mater, pia mater, arachnoid membrane
   E. Pia mater, arachnoid membrane, dura mater

4. Cerebrospinal fluid is normally found predominantly in the
   A. Subdural space
   B. Epidural space
   C. Subarachnoid space
   D. Subpial space

5. Components of the central nervous system include the
   A. Brain and spinal nerves
   B. Spinal nerves and spinal cord
   C. Cranial nerves and brain
   D. Spinal cord and brain

6. The portion of the brain that is largely responsible for coordinating skilled movements, posture, and equilibrium is the
   A. Cerebral cortex
   B. Medulla oblongata
   C. Cerebellum
   D. Spinal cord

7. The physical examination finding that your patient's eyes appear not to move in unison is known as
   A. Doll's eyes
   B. Battle's sign
   C. Disconjugate gaze
   D. Kussmaul's sign

8. Causes of an altered mental state may include
   1. Diabetes mellitus
   2. CNS infection
   3. Illicit drug ingestion
   4. Cerebrovascular accident

A. 1, 2, and 3 are correct
B. 1 and 3 are correct
C. 2 and 4 are correct
D. Only 4 is correct
E. All are correct

9. During your physical examination you note that your patient's neck stiffens when you attempt to flex it. This response is known as
   A. Cervical spondylitis
   B. Homman's sign
   C. Cervical adenopathy
   D. Nuchal rigidity

10. The portion of your physical examination which yields the most diagnostic information about this patient is the
    A. Cardiovascular examination
    B. Neurologic examination
    C. Pulmonary examination
    D. Musculoskeletal examination

11. Abnormal findings encountered in your patient during the neurologic examination include all of the following except
    A. Slurred speech
    B. Disconjugate gaze
    C. Bilateral plantar extension
    D. Nuchal rigidity

12. Your patient's stiff neck in response to attempted flexion suggests
    A. Acute pulmonary embolism
    B. Drug overdose
    C. Classical cerebrovascular accident
    D. Meningitis

13. An infection confined to the lining membranes of the brain and spinal cord is known as
    A. Meningitis
    B. Pleuritis
    C. Encephalitis
    D. Phlebitis

14. An infectious process confined to the brain itself is known as
    A. Meningitis
    B. Pleuritis
    C. Encephalitis
    D. Phlebitis

15. Infectious agents which may cause either meningitis or encephalitis include
    1. Bacteria
    2. Fungi
    3. Viruses
    4. Amoebas

    A. 1, 2, and 3 are correct
    B. 1 and 3 are correct
    C. 2 and 4 are correct
    D. Only 4 is correct
    E. All are correct

16. The findings of fever, an acute change in mental status, and a stiff neck in your patient suggest a field diagnosis of
    A. Acute pulmonary emboli
    B. Cervical spine fracture
    C. Meningitis
    D. Pneumonia
    E. A hypoglycemic event

17. Your patient indicates some reluctance about going to the hospital. His girlfriend is concerned and asks your advice. The most appropriate recommendation would be that
    A. Transport to a hospital is vital so that further evaluation can be carried out
    B. Monitoring of your patient at home over the next day or two is satisfactory
    C. An analgesic such as acetaminophen should be self-administered; if improvement does not occur, she should call back
    D. All of the above are equally advisable

18. Field treatment of your patient should include
    1. Administration of supplemental oxygen
    2. Establishment of a peripheral intravenous line with D5/W
    3. Intravenous administration of thiamine, 50 mg, dextrose, 50 g, and naloxone, 0.4 mg
    4. Sedation with diazepam, 10 mg IV slow push

    A. 1, 2, and 3 are correct
    B. 1 and 3 are correct
    C. 2 and 4 are correct
    D. Only 4 is correct
    E. All are correct

19. Your patient's initial cardiac rhythm (Figure 3–1) is best classified as
    A. Normal sinus rhythm
    B. Sinus tachycardia
    C. Sinus tachycardia with a premature atrial contraction
    D. Sinus tachycardia with a premature ventricular contraction

20. Treatment of your patient's initial cardiac rhythm (Figure 3-1) calls for
    A. Administration of atropine, 0.5 mg IV
    B. Administration of lidocaine, 50 mg IV bolus, followed by a 2 to 4 mg/ml infusion
    C. Administration of verapamil, 5 mg IV slow push
    D. Treatment of underlying cause and continuation of cardiac monitoring (medication is not necessary)

21. Correct statements about bacterial meningitis include
    1. It is a life-threatening condition
    2. Direct exposure to any patient with meningitis requires immediate treatment of the exposed individual
    3. If recognized early it is often effectively treated with antibiotics
    4. It is infrequently seen in infants

    A. 1, 2, and 3 are correct
    B. 1 and 3 are correct
    C. 2 and 4 are correct
    D. Only 4 is correct
    E. All are correct

22. The diagnostic procedure performed in the hospital (Table 3-1) was probably a(n)
    A. Lumbar puncture
    B. Abdominal CT scan
    C. Chest x-ray
    D. Angiography

23. Hospital treatment of bacterial meningitis usually calls for
    A. High dose IV steroids
    B. Low dose radiation therapy
    C. High dose IV antibiotics
    D. Surgical excision and drainage

24. The results of the diagnostic procedure suggest a diagnosis of (Table 3-1)
    A. Acute bacterial meningitis
    B. Acute fungal meningitis
    C. Acute viral meningitis
    D. A hypoglycemic episode

Discussion

Although your patient's clinical presentation is in many respects unremarkable, it does give certain important clues to the underlying disorder. Based on your patient's history and physical examination, the abnormal findings about your patient seem primarily to involve the neurological system. His symptoms include fever, nuchal rigidity, and an altered mental state. Although diabetes mellitus, psychiatric problems, drug ingestion, cerebrovascular accident, head trauma, and several other conditions can all produce an altered mental state, the combination of an altered mental state with fever and nuchal rigidity strongly suggests a diagnosis of meningitis.

Meningitis is an inflammatory process that affects the lining membranes (meninges) of the brain and spinal cord. These membranes, which include the dura mater, arachnoid membrane, and pia mater, (Figure 3–2) may become inflamed in response to neoplastic involvement, contact with irritating chemicals, or contact with an infectious agent. The causative organisms of meningitis due to infection may be bacterial, viral, fungal, or protozoal (Table 3–2). Under certain conditions these organisms may gain entrance to the central nervous system (brain and spinal cord) and result in infection and inflammation. Such an infection may involve the brain tissue, in which case it is termed *encephalitis;* the covering membranes (meninges), in which case it is known as *meningitis;* or both the brain and the overlying meninges, in which case it is referred to as *meningoencephalitis.* Early recognition of meningitis is of utmost importance since the vast majority of infections are amenable to cure through the use of high dose intravenous antibiotics.

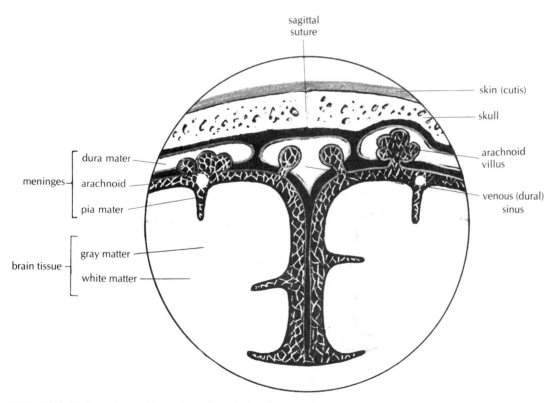

FIGURE 3–2. Frontal section of the head showing meninges and related structures. (Memmler RL, Wood DL: The Human Body in Health and Disease, 6th ed, p 122. Philadelphia, JB Lippincott, 1987)

TABLE 3-2. Causes of Meningitis

Causative Agent	Common Organisms
Bacterial	*Streptococcus pneumonia*
	Neisseria meningitidis
	Staphylococcus aureus
Viral	Coxsackievirus
	Echovirus
	Herpesvirus
Fungal	*Cryptococcus neoformans*
	Coccidioides immitis
	Blastomyces dermatitidis
Protozoal	*Naegleria fowleri*
	Acanthamoeba

Failure to recognize this condition early, however, may lead to rapidly developing cerebral edema, hydrocephalus, increased intracranial pressure, severe neurological damage, or death.

Treatment of this patient should be based on a field diagnosis of an acutely altered mental state, and take into account the fact that his symptoms strongly suggest meningitis. Although a definite diagnosis of meningitis cannot be made in the field, recognizing it as the likely cause of your patient's altered mental state is crucial so that he can immediately be transported to a medical facility and treated with appropriate antibiotic therapy. Although prudent hygienic measures are reasonable in cases of suspected meningitis, most cases are not highly contagious.

After recording vital signs, administer supplemental oxygen and institute cardiac monitoring. Your patient's cardiac rhythm shows an underlying sinus tachycardia at a rate of approximately 110 complexes per minute, with a single premature atrial contraction. Sinus tachycardia frequently occurs in patients with fever of any cause; it is a compensatory mechanism aimed at keeping pace with the increased metabolic activity brought about by elevated body temperature. In view of your patient's stable hemodynamic status and the benign nature of his cardiac arrhythmia, no specific medications need be administered.

Continue monitoring the patient's cardiac rhythm and treating the presenting problem, an altered mental state. Establish a peripheral intravenous (IV) line as a medication route and administer D5/W at a keep-vein-open (KVO) rate. If possible, draw a sample of blood and save it for transport before administering any medications, so that the emergency room physician can determine a medication-free baseline value of your patient's blood components. Three medications that should be administered to treat your patient's marked alteration in mental status are thiamine, dextrose, and naloxone. Although these medications are of little benefit in treating meningitis, it is impossible in the field to be sure that meningitis is the cause of your patient's problem. Hypoglycemia and narcotic ingestion are also frequent causes of altered mental states and are easily corrected by administering these medications. Fifty milligrams of thiamine should be administered as a slow IV bolus, followed by an IV bolus of D50 (50 ml of 50% dextrose). Next, 0.4 mg of naloxone, slow IV bolus, can be administered.

The lack of improvement in your patient's mental status following administration of these medications suggests (though it does not confirm) that neither hypoglycemia nor narcotic ingestion is the primary cause of his altered mental state. Use of sedative or narcotic agents (such as diazepam) is best avoided since they may further alter your patient's mental status, making evaluation difficult if not impossible. Additional management should include frequent monitoring of vital signs, cardiac rhythm, and neurological status.

In cases of suspected meningitis the usual hospital diagnostic procedure is a lumbar puncture ("spinal tap"). This procedure was the one performed on your patient in the emergency room; the results of the test are presented in Table 3-1. A lumbar puncture involves passing a small caliber needle into the spinal canal, usually between the second and third lumbar vertebrae, and removing a sample of the cerebrospinal fluid (CSF). The CSF is then examined microscopically for the presence of organisms (bacteria, fungi, protozoa), analyzed chemically for alterations in levels of protein and glucose, and cultured bacteriologically to see if an infecting organism can be recovered. Its usefulness in cases of suspected meningitis revolves around the fact that very often the CSF of patients with meningitis will show either the presence of the infecting organism, or characteristic changes in the chemical composition of the fluid which allow one to infer the presence of an organism, even if it cannot be directly seen. The results of the analysis of your patient's CSF are remarkable because they show an increased number of leukocytes—specifically polymorphonuclear leukocytes (PMNs)—an increased protein concentration, and a decreased glucose concentration. These findings together suggest an acute meningitis of bacterial origin.

Field Diagnosis
- Altered mental state
- Possible meningitis

Hospital Diagnosis
- Acute bacterial meningitis

Patient Follow-Up

Your patient was admitted to the medical service with a diagnosis of acute bacterial meningitis and treated immediately with IV penicillin. The following day his CSF culture revealed *Streptococcus pneumonia* (a gram-positive organism). Following a successful antibiotic course, your patient recovered without obvious residual damage and was discharged with a recommendation for further follow-up.

Answers

1. **A**
   Caroline NL: Emergency Care in the Streets, 3rd ed, pp 14–30. Boston, Little, Brown & Co, 1987

2. **D**
   Taber's Cyclopedic Medical Dictionary, 14th ed, sv "meninges"

3. **E**
   Caroline NL: Emergency Care in the Streets, 3rd ed, pp 13–56. Boston, Little, Brown & Co, 1987
   Memmler RL, Wood DL: The Human Body in Health and Disease, 5th ed, p 141. Philadelphia, JB Lippincott, 1983

4. **C**
   Caroline NL: Emergency Care in the Streets, 3rd ed, pp 13–56. Boston, Little, Brown & Co, 1987
   American Academy of Orthopaedic Surgeons: Emergency Care and Transportation of the Sick and Injured, 3rd ed, p 179. Menasha, WI, George Banta Co, 1981

5. **D**
   Caroline NL: Emergency Care in the Streets, 3rd ed, pp 13–56. Boston, Little, Brown & Co, 1987
   American Academy of Orthopaedic Surgeons: Emergency Care and Transportation of the Sick and Injured, 3rd ed, p 179. Menasha, WI, George Banta Co, 1981

6. **C**
   Caroline NL: Emergency Care in the Streets, 3rd ed, pp 13–56. Boston, Little, Brown & Co, 1987
   Guyton AC: Textbook of Medical Physiology, 6th ed, pp 658–659. Philadelphia, WB Saunders, 1981

7. **C**
   Caroline NL: Emergency Care in the Streets, 3rd ed, pp 13–56. Boston, Little, Brown & Co, 1987

8. **E**
   Caroline NL: Emergency Care in the Streets, 3rd ed, pp 345–374. Boston, Little, Brown & Co, 1987
   Anderson D, Cosgriff JH Jr: The comatose patient. In Cosgriff JH Jr, Anderson DL: The Practice of Emergency Care, 2nd ed, pp 288–302. Philadelphia, JB Lippincott, 1984

9. **D**
   Taber's Cyclopedic Medical Dictionary, 14th ed, sv "nuchal"

10. **B**
    Swartz MN: Bacterial meningitis. In Wyngaarden JB, Smith LH Jr: Textbook of Medicine, 17th ed, pp 1552–1553. Philadelphia, WB Saunders, 1985

11. **C**
    Bates B: A Guide to Physical Examination, 3rd ed, p 407. Philadelphia, JB Lippincott, 1983
    Delp MH, Manning RT: Major's Physical Diagnosis, 9th ed, pp 109–110. Philadelphia, WB Saunders, 1981

12. **D**
    Caroline NL: Emergency Care in the Streets, 3rd ed, pp 345–374. Boston, Little, Brown & Co, 1987
    Swartz MN: Bacterial meningitis. In Wyngaarden JB, Smith LH Jr: Textbook of Medicine, 17th ed, pp 1552–1553. Philadelphia, WB Saunders, 1985

13. **A**
    American Academy of Orthopaedic Surgeons: Emergency Care and Transportation of the Sick and Injured, 3rd ed, p 179. Menasha, WI, George Banta Co, 1981

14. **C**
    Taber's Cyclopedic Medical Dictionary, 14th ed, sv "meningitis"

15. **E**
    American Academy of Orthopaedic Surgeons: Emergency Care and Transportation of the Sick and Injured, 3rd ed, p 179. Menasha, WI, George Banta Co, 1981
    Krogstad DJ: Amebiasis and amebic meningoencephalitis. In Wyngaarden JB, Smith LH Jr: Textbook of Medicine, 17th ed, p 1801. Philadelphia, WB Saunders, 1985

16. **C**
    Caroline NL: Emergency Care in the Streets, 3rd ed, pp 345–74. Boston, Little, Brown & Co, 1987
    American Academy of Orthopaedic Surgeons: Emergency Care and Transportation of the Sick and Injured, 3rd ed, p 179. Menasha, WI, George Banta Co, 1981

17. A

   Swartz MN: Bacterial meningitis. In Wyngaarden JB, Smith LH Jr: Textbook of Medicine, 17th ed, p 1555. Philadelphia, WB Saunders, 1985

18. A

   Caroline NL: Emergency Care in the Streets, 3rd ed, pp 345–374. Boston, Little, Brown & Co, 1987

19. C

   Huff J, Doernbach DP, White RD: ECG Workout: Exercises in Arrhythmia Interpretation, pp 49, 220 (strip 2.21). Philadelphia, JB Lippincott, 1985

20. D

   Caroline NL: Emergency Care in the Streets, 3rd ed, pp 251–344. Boston, Little, Brown & Co, 1987
   Huszar RJ: Emergency Cardiac Care, pp 134–135. Bowie, MD, Robert J Brady Co, 1974

21. B

   Swartz MN: Bacterial meningitis. In Wyngaarden JB, Smith LH Jr: Textbook of Medicine, 17th ed, pp 1551–1556. Philadelphia, WB Saunders, 1985

22. A

   Anderson D, Cosgriff JH Jr: The comatose patient. In Cosgriff JH Jr, Anderson DL: The Practice of Emergency Care, 2nd ed, p 293. Philadelphia, JB Lippincott, 1984
   Plum F: The neurologic examination. In Wyngaarden JB, Smith LH Jr: Textbook of Medicine, 17th ed, pp 1968–1969. Philadelphia, WB Saunders, 1985

23. C

   Swartz MN: Bacterial meningitis. In Wyngaarden JB, Smith LH Jr: Textbook of Medicine, 17th ed, pp 1555–1556. Philadelphia, WB Saunders, 1985
   Hoffman TA: Purulent bacterial meningitis. In Braude AI (ed): Medical Microbiology and Infectious Disease, pp 1237–1238. Philadelphia, WB Saunders, 1981

24. A

   Hoffman TA: Purulent bacterial meningitis. In Braude AI (ed): Medical Microbiology and Infectious Disease, p 1237. Philadelphia, WB Saunders, 1981
   Swartz MN: Bacterial meningitis. In Wyngaarden JB, Smith LH Jr: Textbook of Medicine, 17th ed., p 1553. Philadelphia, WB Saunders, 1985

Selected Reading

Hoffman TA: Purulent bacterial meningitis. In Braude AI (ed): Medical Microbiology and Infectious Disease, pp 1234–1239. Philadelphia, WB Saunders, 1981

Carpenter RR, Petersdorf RG: The clinical spectrum of bacterial meningitis. Am J Med 33:262, 1962

Swartz MN: Intracranial infections. In Rosenberg RN (ed): The Science and Practice of Clinical Medicine, Vol 5. New York, Grune & Stratton, 1980

4

Dyspnea and Rash in a Young Woman

Your ambulance is called for a priority one job and requested to report to an Oriental restaurant to aid a woman with "difficulty breathing." When you arrive at the scene you are directed to your patient, who is an agitated young woman in marked respiratory distress, using accessory muscles for respiration. No definite stridor is heard and your patient is able to tell you her full name.

Your patient denies medication use as well as any other medical history. She also vehemently denies intravenous drug use. Vital signs at this time are BP (right arm, sitting) 80/40, pulse 130 regular and thready, respiration 26 and labored, and temperature cool to touch.

Your patient is a 22-year-old woman with a pallid appearance weighing approximately 110 pounds. She is alert and oriented and responds to commands. Pupils are round, equal, and reactive to light. Throat, pharynx, and oropharynx are clear of foreign objects. The trachea is midline and easily mobile and carotid pulses are equal. Most notable immediately is a wheal-like rash that is spreading over the trunk, extremities, and face. Anterior and posterior thoracic examination reveals adequate excursion without splinting. Auscultation reveals adequate air exchange, although diffuse bilateral inspiratory wheezes are heard. Heart sounds are normal S_1 S_2, although obscured by the wheezes. The point of maximal impulse (PMI) is normally placed and no jugular venous distension (JVD) is present with the patient inclined at a 45-degree angle. Pedal edema and clubbing are absent.

Intravenous (IV) access is obtained and 10 ml of 1:10,000 dilution of an appropriate medication are administered. Your patient's cardiac rhythm is monitored (Figure 4-1) and transport begins. Vital signs include BP (left arm, sitting) 70 by palpation, and your patient shows signs of increasing laryngeal edema and some lethargy. You contact medical control and they approve a repeat dose of medication. A second IV line is placed. Both are now running at maximal drip rate. Medical control grants approval to use a pressor agent if the patient does not respond to fluids. Because you note increasing stridor, you request that otolaryngology and anesthesiology services stand by at the emergency room. For the remainder of transport your patient's vital signs are BP (left arm, sitting) 110/70, pulse 130 regular and weak, and respiration 24 regular and labored. She shows continued signs of laryngeal edema and stridor. Another rhythm strip is recorded (Figure 4-2).

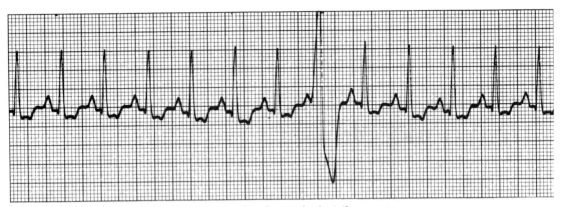

FIGURE 4-1. Lead II EKG recorded shortly after arrival at the scene.

When you arrive at the emergency room, the patient's condition is immediately evaluated by medical, otolaryngology, and anesthesiology services. Blood is drawn for chemical analysis, further medications are administered, and an arterial blood gas (ABG) evaluation is performed. A stat 12 lead EKG and chest radiograph are ordered.

Questions

Read each question carefully, keeping in mind the context of the case under discussion. Select the best answer from the choices presented.

1. In view of your patient's clinical condition, the best working field diagnosis is
   A. Anaphylactic shock
   B. Cardiogenic shock
   C. Neurogenic shock
   D. Acute pulmonary edema

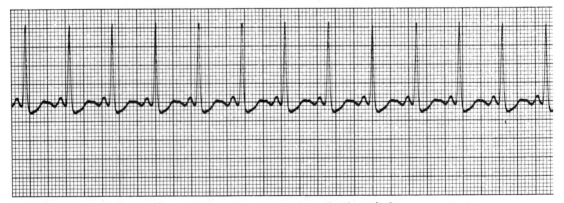

FIGURE 4-2. Lead II EKG recorded during transport to the hospital.

2. The etiology of your patient's condition is best classified as
   A. Infectious
   B. Allergic
   C. Ischemic
   D. Toxic

3. Initial field treatment of your patient should include
   1. Establishment of an intravenous line
   2. Immediate intubation
   3. Application of MAST
   4. Performance of a cricothyroidotomy

   A. 1, 2, and 3 are correct
   B. 1 and 3 are correct
   C. 2 and 4 are correct
   D. Only 4 is correct
   E. All are correct

4. The appropriate medication approved initially by medical control and administered IV as 10 ml of 1:10,000 dilution was most probably
   A. Dopamine
   B. Isoproterenol
   C. Atropine
   D. Epinephrine

5. The most useful clue in helping you to determine the cause of your patient's condition is
   A. Hypotension
   B. Wheezing
   C. A fleeting urticarial rash
   D. Dyspnea

6. The intravenous fluid of choice in this case is
   A. D5/W
   B. D5/normal saline
   C. Packed red blood cells
   D. Whole fresh blood

7. An important reason for requesting an ENT standby is that
   A. Your patient may require insertion of a chest tube
   B. Intubation must be carried out using an EOA, which is best placed by an ENT specialist
   C. There is a possibility that laryngeal edema may require a difficult intubation or a tracheotomy
   D. Your patient has abnormally aspirated a foreign body and its removal will require using Magill forceps

8. Should your patient's blood pressure continue to decline, an intravenous infusion of which of the following medications is likely to be most valuable?
   A. Dopamine or norepinephrine
   B. Norepinephrine or diphenhydramine (Benadryl)
   C. Propranolol or dopamine
   D. Diphenhydramine (Benadryl) or atropine

9. Which of the following medications possesses the greatest β-agonistic properties?
   A. Propranolol
   B. Phenylephrine
   C. Epinephrine
   D. Aminophylline

10. Drugs used to minimize pulmonary bronchospasm are most likely to possess
    A. α-antagonistic properties
    B. β-agonistic properties
    C. α-agonistic properties
    D. β-antagonistic properties

11. Peripheral vasoconstriction most commonly occurs with drugs that possess
    A. β-antagonistic properties
    B. α-agonistic properties
    C. β-agonistic properties
    D. α-antagonistic properties

12. Aminophylline may be useful in treating your patient because of its
    A. Potent diuretic effects
    B. Anti-arrhythmogenic effects
    C. Vasoconstrictive effects
    D. Bronchodilatory effects

13. Which of the following choices represents an incorrect medication dosage and route?
    A. Aminophylline 6 mg/kg, slow IV drip, over 30 minutes
    B. Dopamine infusion at 2 to 5 ug/kg/min
    C. Epinephrine 1:1,000 solution, IV bolus
    D. Diphenhydramine (Benadryl) 25 mg, IV push or IM

14. Oxygen therapy for your patient is best carried out using a
    A. Nasal cannula at 1 to 2 l/m
    B. Venturi mask at 24%
    C. Non-rebreathing face mask at 6 to 8 l/m
    D. Rebreathing face mask at 4 l/m

15. Which of the following conditions may present with laryngeal edema and respiratory distress?

1. Anaphylactic shock
2. Hereditary angioneurotic edema
3. Bacterial epiglottitis
4. Inhalational injuries

A. 1, 2, and 3 are correct
B. 1 and 3 are correct
C. 2 and 4 are correct
D. Only 4 is correct
E. All are correct

16. The cardiac rhythm shown in Figure 4-1 is correctly classified as
    A. Normal sinus rhythm
    B. Second degree AV block with a premature atrial contraction
    C. Paroxysmal atrial tachycardia
    D. Sinus tachycardia with a premature ventricular contraction

17. The rhythm shown in Figure 4-1 is best managed by
    A. Administration of lidocaine, 100 mg IV bolus, followed by a 2 to 4 mg/min infusion
    B. Administration of bretylium tosylate, 5 to 6 mg IV push, followed by an infusion
    C. Supportive measures only; correction of underlying condition
    D. Defibrillation at 360 J

18. Which of the following sets of medications is likely to be most useful in treating your patient?
    A. Norepinephrine—propranolol—diphenhydramine (Benadryl)—dexamethasone
    B. Epinephrine—dexamethasone—aminophylline—diphenhydramine (Benadryl)
    C. Isoproterenol—aminophylline—calcium chloride—naloxone
    D. Epinephrine—aminophylline—diphenhydramine (Benadryl)—morphine sulfate

19. Factors which may precipitate the clinical condition seen in your patient include
    1. Bee sting
    2. Penicillin
    3. Seafood
    4. Aspirin

    A. 1, 2, and 3 are correct
    B. 1 and 3 are correct
    C. 2 and 4 are correct
    D. Only 4 is correct
    E. All are correct

20. Your patient's cardiac rhythm recorded during transport to the hospital (Figure 4-2) is best classified as
    A. Sinus tachycardia
    B. Normal sinus rhythm
    C. Sinus bradycardia
    D. Atrial fibrillation

Discussion

Your patient's symptoms—hypotension, tachycardia, diaphoresis, and pallor—suggest early manifestations of shock (see "Signs and Symptoms of Shock"). *Shock* may be defined as a pathophysiological state having multiple etiologies, the common denominator of which is inadequate tissue perfusion. It is vital to recognize and diagnose shock early as well as to determine its etiology, because prognosis depends on appropriate and early aggressive medical management. Shock states may be classified according to five basic types: *cardiogenic, neurogenic, septic, toxic-metabolic,* and *anaphylactic.* Despite their differing etiologies, all five types have in common the presenting symptoms of hypotension, tachycardia, and diaphoresis. Any patient with this symptomatology should be evaluated for the possibility of underlying shock. Because the signs and symptoms of the different forms are often similar, the clinical history may help to elucidate the etiology of the shock state.

For this patient, a diagnosis of cardiogenic shock would be most unlikely in view of the patient's young age, sex, negative past medical history, and most importantly, lack of antecedent chest pain. Neurogenic shock is unlikely because there is no report of recent trauma, medication ingestion, or insect bites. The finding of a rapid heart rate (tachycardia) in this patient also argues against the possibility of neurogenic shock, since this is one of the few forms of shock often characterized by a slow pulse rate (bradycardia) due to interference with the sympathetic nerve supply to the heart.

Toxic-metabolic shock is also unlikely in the absence of any identifiable predisposing medical condition, such as diabetes mellitus, uremia, or drug ingestion. Although the possibility of septic shock must always be entertained in any case of unexplained hypotension, the lack of supporting factors, such as fever, chills, or a recent history of infection, makes this diagnosis improbable. The remaining possibility is anaphylactic shock. Your patient's signs (hypotension, tachycardia, and diaphoresis), in addition to the findings of a spreading wheal-like

---

Signs and Symptoms of Shock

Altered mental state
Cool, clammy, pale skin
Rapid, weak pulse
Increased respiratory rate
Hypotension
Diaphoresis

Common Agents Causing Anaphylaxis
Penicillin
Tetracycline
Aspirin
Seafood
Insect stings

rash, laryngeal edema, and bronchospasm in relation to ingesting food that is known to be allergenic in some individuals, point instead to anaphylactic shock as the cause of your patient's problem.

Anaphylactic shock is a generalized reaction to an inciting allergen which causes the release of several chemical mediators into the blood stream (see "Common Agents Causing Anaphylaxis"). These mediators in turn cause hypotension, laryngeal edema and stridor, bronchospasm and wheezing, and urticarial rash ("hives"). Although clinical presentation varies, when all these symptoms exist the condition is life threatening. It is therefore imperative to recognize and aggressively treat anaphylactic shock in its early stages.

The basic goals of treatment are maintaining a patent airway, correcting significant bronchospasm, and reversing vascular collapse (see "Treatment of Anaphylactic Shock"). Initial treatment should include measures to ensure an open and patent airway and adequate oxygenation. If complete airway closure has occurred owing to laryngeal edema, a cricothyroidotomy is indicated, if this procedure is within the provider's scope of training and local operating protocols. If complete airway closure has not occurred but marked respiratory failure is present, immediate endotracheal intubation and ventilatory assistance may be necessary. In the present case, the patient's respiratory status, although somewhat compromised, does not warrant such aggressive measures. Instead, using high concentration humidified oxygen and careful airway monitoring are called for.

Hemodynamic stabilization should be carried out because the patient's initial blood pressure (80/40) indicates an effectively hypovolemic state. Establish a peripheral intravenous (IV) line and apply military antishock trousers (MAST) (inflate if vital signs and local protocols require). Fluid replacement should be accomplished by rapid infusion of a crystalloid solution such as normal saline or lactated Ringer's.

Treatment of Anaphylactic Shock

- Establish a patent airway
- Monitor vital signs
- Monitor cardiac rhythm
- Establish an intravenous line
- In consultation with medical control consider administration of:
    Epinephrine: For moderate anaphylactic reaction, 0.3–0.5 ml of 1:1,000 dilution SC. For severe anaphylactic reaction, 5–10 ml of 1:10,000 dilution, slow IV push
    Aminophylline: 6 mg/kg by IV infusion given over 20–40 minutes
    Diphenhydramine: 10–50 mg slow IV push or deep IM
    Dexamethasone: 4 mg, slow IV injection

Medications which may be useful in treating anaphylactic shock include epinephrine, aminophylline, vasopressors (norepinephrine and dopamine), diphenhydramine (Benadryl), and steroids (*eg,* hydrocortisone). Epinephrine is the first line drug of choice for anaphylactic shock. Depending on the severity of the patient's condition, it may be administered either subcutaneously as 0.5 ml of a 1:1,000 solution or intravenously as 5 to 10 ml of a 1:10,000 solution. Its therapeutic effects are complex but include moderating the release of toxic anaphylactic mediators, lessening laryngeal edema, and a beneficial bronchodilatory effect.

Aminophylline, a methylxanthine, is valuable in cases of anaphylaxis because of its marked ability to relax bronchial smooth muscle, thereby relieving bronchospasm and improving ventilation. The most serious side-effects associated with aminophylline include hypotension, cardiac arrhythmias, and seizures. Because these effects are more likely to occur as a result of either rapid administration or high plasma levels, it is important that aminophylline be administered slowly and at the lowest dose necessary to produce the desired effects. This approach is best achieved by setting up an aminophylline infusion with a loading dose of 6 mg/kg administered over 20 to 40 minutes. Since the patient under consideration has an approximate body weight of 50 kg, the total dose of medication should be 300 mg (6 mg/kg $\times$ 50 kg). In order to administer this quantity over a period of approximately 30 minutes, a reasonable approach would be first to add the contents of one 500 mg ampule of aminophylline to 250 ml of D5/W, yielding a solution with a concentration of 2 mg/ml. Administering 150 ml of this solution will deliver the total desired dose of 300 mg of aminophylline (150 ml $\times$ 2 mg aminophylline/ml). Using an infusion set which delivers 10 drops/ml, one can administer the entire 300 mg dose of medication over a period of 30 minutes by adjusting the drip rate to 50 drops per minute. A clearly marked label indicating the date and paramedic's name, name of the medication, amount of medication added, resulting concentration, time at which the infusion was started, and set time, if any, at which the patient will have received the full therapeutic dose, should be attached to the intravenous bag.

Diphenhydramine (Benadryl) acts as a histamine antagonist and is the prototype of a class of drugs known as antihistamines. Endogenous histamine is one of the several chemical mediators released by the body during anaphylaxis that bring about the life-threatening reactions associated with systemic anaphylaxis. By blocking some of the effects of histamine, diphenhydramine may help to relieve some of the symptoms of anaphylaxis. Because the more serious complications of anaphylaxis, such as hypotension and bronchoconstriction, are largely mediated by released substances other than histamine, however, such agents as diphenhydramine are only minimally effective in treating the more serious consequences of anaphylaxis. An antihistamine should therefore be used only as an adjunct with a more effective drug such as epinephrine. Diphenhydramine is usually administered either intramuscularly or intravenously in doses of between 10 and 50 mg.

Steroids, specifically glucocorticosteroids, are a group of compounds which includes hydrocortisone (Solu-Cortef), methylprednisolone (Solu-Medrol), and dexamethasone (Decadron). These agents may help, by an incompletely understood mechanism, in the management of anaphylaxis. Like antihistamines, these medications should play only a supportive role. The mainstay of therapy for acute systemic anaphylaxis must consist of more effective agents.

Finally, if your patient remains hypotensive after receiving fluids and the above medications, the use of vasopressor agents such as dopamine or norepinephrine may be indicated. In the present case your patient shows signs of hemodynamic improvement after receiving fluids and epinephrine. Respiratory distress, however, is still evident. Because the possibility of complete airway closure secondary to laryngeal edema is real, the decision to request an ENT and anesthesiology standby is warranted.

Field Diagnosis
- Shock, probably secondary to anaphylaxis

Hospital Diagnosis
- Anaphylactic shock

Patient Follow-Up

After arriving at the emergency room your patient was given 200 mg hydrocortisone IV, diphenhydramine, 50 mg IV, and nebulizer treatment. Her airway was believed to be patent by both ENT and anesthesiology. Laryngeal edema gradually decreased. She was admitted to the floor for observation and a careful history was taken in an attempt to identify the inciting agent. Vital signs remained stable and the following day she was released, with follow-up to be conducted in the allergy clinic.

Answers

1. A
   Caroline NL: Emergency Care in the Streets, 3rd ed, pp 424–425. Boston, Little, Brown & Co, 1987
   Lichtenstein LM: Anaphylaxis. In Wyngaarden JB, Smith LH Jr: Textbook of Medicine, 17th ed, pp 1870–1872. Philadelphia, WB Saunders, 1985

2. B
   Caroline NL: Emergency Care in the Streets, 3rd ed, pp 424–425. Boston, Little, Brown & Co, 1987
   Lichtenstein LM: Anaphylaxis. In Wyngaarden JB, Smith LH Jr: Textbook of Medicine, 17th ed, pp 1870–1872. Philadelphia, WB Saunders 1985

3. B
   Caroline NL: Emergency Care in the Streets, 3rd ed, pp 424–425. Boston, Little, Brown & Co, 1987
   Anderson D, Cosgriff JH Jr: Bites and stings. In Cosgriff JH Jr, Anderson DL: The Practice of Emergency Care, 2nd ed, pp 562–563. Philadelphia, JB Lippincott, 1984

4. D
   Caroline NL: Emergency Care in the Streets, 3rd ed, pp 424–425. Boston, Little, Brown & Co, 1987
   Anderson D, Cosgriff JH Jr: Bites and stings. In Cosgriff JH Jr, Anderson DL: The Practice of Emergency Care, 2nd ed, p 563. Philadelphia, JB Lippincott, 1984

5. C
   Caroline NL: Emergency Care in the Streets, 3rd ed, pp 424–425. Boston, Little, Brown & Co, 1987
   Soter NA, Wasserman SI: IgE-Dependent urticaria, angioedema, and anaphylaxis. In Fitzpatrick TB, Eisen AZ, Wolff K (eds): Dermatology in General Medicine, 2nd ed, pp 534, 538. New York, McGraw-Hill, 1979

6. B
   Caroline NL: Emergency Care in the Streets, 3rd ed, pp 424–425. Boston, Little, Brown & Co, 1987
   Baldwin L, Pierce R: Mobile Intensive Care: A Problem-Oriented Approach, p 261. St Louis, CV Mosby, 1978

7. C
   Lichtenstein LM: Anaphylaxis. In Wyngaarden JB, Smith LH Jr: Textbook of Medicine, 17th ed, p 1871. Philadelphia, WB Saunders, 1985

8. A
   Caroline NL: Emergency Care in the Streets, 3rd ed, pp 424–425. Boston, Little, Brown & Co, 1987

9. C
   Caroline NL: Emergency Care in the Streets, 3rd ed, pp 112–119. Boston, Little, Brown & Co, 1987
   Weiner N: Norepinephrine, epinephrine, and the sympathomimetic amines. In Gilman AG, Goodman LS, Rall TW (eds): The Pharmacological Basis of Therapeutics, 7th ed, pp 145–158. New York, Macmillan, 1985

10. B
    Caroline NL: Emergency Care in the Streets, 3rd ed, pp 112–119. Boston, Little, Brown & Co, 1987
    Hoffman BB: Adrenergic receptor-activating drugs. In Katzung BG (ed): Basic and Clinical Pharmacology, pp 72–81. Los Altos, Lange Medical Publications, 1982

11. B
    Caroline NL: Emergency Care in the Streets, 3rd ed, pp 112–119. Boston, Little, Brown & Co, 1987
    Hoffman BB: Adrenergic receptor-activating drugs. In Katzung BG (ed): Basic and Clinical Pharmacology, pp 72–81. Los Altos, Lange Medical Publications, 1982

12. D
    Rall TW: Central nervous system stimulants. In Gilman AG, Goodman LS, Rall TW (eds): The Pharmacological Basis of Therapeutics, 7th ed, pp 589–601. New York, Macmillan, 1985

13. C
    Caroline NL: Emergency Care in the Streets, 3rd ed, pp 130–141. Boston, Little, Brown & Co, 1987

14. C
    Baldwin L, Pierce R: Mobile Intensive Care: A Problem-Oriented Approach, p 262. St Louis, CV Mosby, 1978
    Anderson D, Cosgriff JH Jr.: Bites and stings. In Cosgriff JH Jr, Anderson DL: The Practice of Emergency Care, 2nd ed, pp 562–563. Philadelphia, JB Lippincott, 1984

15. E
    Caroline NL: Emergency Care in the Streets, 3rd ed, pp 424–425. Boston, Little, Brown & Co, 1987
    Fearon DT: Complement. In Wyngaarden JB, Smith LH Jr: Textbook of Medicine, 17th ed, p 1854. Philadelphia, WB Saunders, 1985

16. D
    Huff J, Doernbach DP, White RD: ECG Workout: Exercises in Arrhythmia Interpretation, pp 140, 241 (strip 4.66). Philadelphia, JB Lippincott, 1985
    Alpert MA: Cardiac Arrhythmias, pp 8–10, 17–33. Chicago, Year Book Medical Publishers, 1980

17. C
    Caroline NL: Emergency Care in the Streets, 3rd ed, p 297. Boston, Little, Brown & Co, 1987
    Alpert MA: Cardiac Arrhythmias, p 31. Chicago, Year Book Medical Publishers, 1980
    Walraven G, Harding J, Leblanc KM et al: Manual of Advanced Prehospital Care, pp 262–263. Bowie, MD, Robert J Brady Co, 1978

18. B
    Caroline NL: Emergency Care in the Streets, 3rd ed, pp 424–425. Boston, Little, Brown & Co, 1987
    Walraven G, Harding J, Leblanc KM et al: Manual of Advanced Prehospital Care. pp 87, 153. Bowie, MD, Robert J Brady Co, 1978

19. E

Caroline NL: Emergency Care in the Streets, 3rd ed, pp 424–425. Boston, Little, Brown & Co, 1987

Lichtenstein LM: Anaphylaxis. In Wyngaarden JB, Smith LH Jr: Textbook of Medicine, 17th ed, p 1871. Philadelphia, WB Saunders, 1985

20. A

Huff J, Doernbach DP, White RD: ECG Workout: Exercises in Arrhythmia Interpretation, pp 33, 218 (strip 1.83). Philadelphia, JB Lippincott, 1985

Selected Reading

Lichtenstein LM: Anaphylaxis. In Wyngaarden JB, Smith LH Jr: Textbook of Medicine, 17th ed, pp. 1870–1872. Philadelphia, WB Saunders, 1985

5

A Syncopal Episode in a Chronic Alcoholic

Your dispatcher calls, notifying you of a person experiencing a "syncopal episode" in your response area. Arriving at your patient's residence, you find him lying on the floor. He is conscious, but confused and lethargic. The family reports that they were upstairs when they heard a loud noise and, descending, discovered him supine. Further questioning reveals that for the past two days your patient's stools have been tarry-black and foul-smelling, and that yesterday he complained of lightheadedness. Your patient denies any chest pain, shortness of breath, chills, or fever. He does, however, admit that he has had palpitations both last night and today.

Past medical history includes chronic alcoholism, pancreatitis, and hepatitis two years prior. Medications include multivitamins, 1 tablet po od, and thiamine, 100 mg po od. Your patient denies any use of aspirin or aspirin-containing substances and any recent alcohol intake. He reports that he is allergic to penicillin (he broke out in a diffuse rash and experienced generalized body swelling the last time it was administered).

Your patient is a 51-year-old man who, though conscious, is somewhat difficult to arouse. Vital signs are BP (right arm, recumbent) 120/90, pulse 124 regular and weak, respiration 24 and regular, and temperature cool to touch. Rechecked with your patient sitting erect, vital signs are BP (right arm, sitting) 80 by palpation, and pulse 142 regular and thready. His head and neck show no signs of trauma. His trachea is midline and mobile and his neck is supple. A patent airway is present and free of foreign matter, although halitosis is detected. Conjunctiva are markedly pale and the sclera appear icteric. Lung examination reveals a few scattered rhonchi, but adequate breath sounds are heard bilaterally, and respiratory excursion is symmetrical. Heart sounds are S_1S_2, though increased in intensity, with a systolic murmur heard best at the base of the heart. No gallop sounds are noted. Jugular venous distension (JVD) is present with the patient inclined at a 45-degree angle.

Abdominal examination reveals a scaphoid abdomen and increased frequency of bowel sounds. The abdomen is soft and nontender although a nonpulsatile, firm mass is palpated in the upper left abdominal quadrant. A fluid wave is not elicited and the flanks are not bulging. Extremities show 2 plus pitting pedal edema, and poor capillary refill in both the upper and lower nail beds is noted. Neurologic examination shows a conscious, though lethargic, individual oriented only to person. Pupils are round, equal, and reactive to light. No gross focal findings are noted.

Field treatment is instituted immediately while medical control is contacted. Your patient's vital signs at this time are BP (right arm, recumbent) 120/80, pulse 136 regular and weak, respiration 24, and temperature cool to touch. His initial cardiac rhythm is shown in Figure 5-1. Transport begins and a notification is requested. Five minutes into transport your patient starts to experience severe nausea and promptly vomits 200 to 300 ml of fresh red blood. His vital signs are measured again: BP (right arm, supine) 110/72, pulse 136 irregular and weak, respiration 26 and regular, and temperature cool to touch. After conferring with medical control, you administer a colloidal volume expander. A dopamine drip is also prepared and held in reserve, in case the systolic pressure continues to fall below 80 mm Hg despite aggressive fluid replacement. Your patient remains alert and continues to deny any chest pain.

Upon arrival at the hospital, you are greeted by medical and nursing personnel, and further medical management, including immediate transfusion of saline cross-matched blood, is undertaken. A spun hematocrit taken in the emergency room is 12%.

Questions

Read each question carefully, keeping in mind the context of the case under discussion. Select the best answer from the choices presented.

1. The passage of tarry-black, foul-smelling stools by your patient is known as
   A. Melena
   B. Hematemesis
   C. Myoglobin
   D. Hematuria

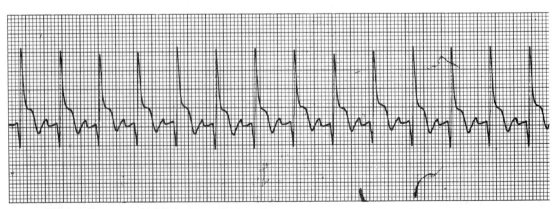

FIGURE 5-1. Lead II EKG recorded shortly after arrival.

2. Tarry-black, foul-smelling stools are associated with
    A. Gastrointestinal bleeding
    B. External hemorrhage
    C. Genitourinary hemorrhage
    D. Acute appendicitis

3. A history of chronic alcoholism (as in the case of your patient) is associated with which of the following?
    1. Pancreatitis
    2. Acute appendicitis
    3. Cirrhosis
    4. Cor pulmonale

    A. 1, 2, and 3 are correct
    B. 1 and 3 are correct
    C. 2 and 4 are correct
    D. Only 4 is correct
    E. All are correct

4. Expected findings in a patient suffering from liver disease secondary to chronic alcoholism include all the following except
    A. Ascites
    B. Jaundice
    C. Peripheral edema
    D. Acute pulmonary edema

5. The differences noted in your patient's blood pressure and pulse when he is moved from a supine to a sitting position are known as
    A. Pulse deficit
    B. Epistaxis
    C. Hypostatic changes
    D. Orthostatic changes

6. The above finding in your patient suggests
    A. Acute myocardial infarction
    B. Intravascular volume depletion
    C. Acute alcohol intoxication
    D. Underlying diabetes mellitus

7. Pitting pedal edema may be due to
    1. Decreased arterial pressure
    2. Hypoalbuminemia
    3. Hyperalbuminemia
    4. Increased systemic venous pressure

    A. 1, 2, and 3 are correct
    B. 1 and 3 are correct
    C. 2 and 4 are correct

Medical Emergencies

    D. Only 4 is correct
    E. All are correct

8. Your physical examination reveals a systolic heart murmur. By definition this implies an occurrence
    A. Between S_1 and S_2
    B. Starting with S_1 and continuing until the following S_1
    C. Between S_2 and S_1
    D. Starting with S_2 and continuing until the following S_2

9. The firm nonpulsatile abdominal mass palpated in the upper left quadrant is most probably the
    A. Gallbladder
    B. Pancreas
    C. Spleen
    D. Appendix

10. Which of the following conditions, when accompanied by blood loss, is not considered an upper gastrointestinal bleed?
    A. Gastritis
    B. Duodenal ulcer
    C. Esophageal varices
    D. Colonic perforation

11. The best field diagnosis for this patient is that of a(n)
    A. Perforated duodenal ulcer
    B. Upper gastrointestinal bleed
    C. Hemothorax
    D. Ruptured abdominal aortic aneurysm
    E. Lower gastrointestinal bleed

12. Initial field treatment of your patient calls for
    1. Placement of two large-bore intravenous lines and rapid infusion of fluid
    2. Immediate endotracheal intubation
    3. Application and inflation of MAST
    4. Carotid sinus massage

    A. 1, 2, and 3 are correct
    B. 1 and 3 are correct
    C. 2 and 4 are correct
    D. Only 4 is correct
    E. All are correct

13. Initial medications that may be useful for treating your patient include
    1. D50, IV bolus
    2. Thiamine, 50 mg IV slow push
    3. Naloxone, 0.4 mg IV bolus
    4. Dopamine infusion 12 ug/kg/min

A. 1, 2, and 3 are correct
B. 1 and 3 are correct
C. 2 and 4 are correct
D. Only 4 is correct
E. All are correct

14. During transport a decision is made in consultation with medical control to administer a colloidal volume expander to counteract your patient's continued hemodynamic deterioration. Which of the following fluids are you likely to use?
    A. Human plasma protein fraction (Plasmanate)
    B. D5/W
    C. Lactated Ringer's
    D. 3% normal saline

15. In comparison with crystalloid volume expanders, colloidal volume expanders show a greater ability to
    A. Bind and transport oxygen
    B. Expand the intracellular fluid
    C. Remain within the intravascular compartment
    D. Function as a metabolic energy source

16. The life-threatening complication seen most commonly in association with chronic alcoholism is
    A. Alcohol withdrawal seizures
    B. Dissecting aortic aneurysm
    C. Acute pulmonary edema
    D. Esophageal varices

17. Your patient's initial cardiac rhythm (Figure 5-1) is best classified as
    A. Normal sinus rhythm
    B. Atrial tachycardia
    C. Ventricular tachycardia
    D. Sinus tachycardia

18. The pigment that is responsible for the scleral icterus seen in your patient is
    A. Myoglobin
    B. Bilirubin
    C. Hemoglobin
    D. Melanin

19. Regarding the term "gastrointestinal bleed," which of the following statements are correct?
    1. An upper gastrointestinal bleed has a primary site of blood loss above the ligament of Treitz
    2. A lower gastrointestinal bleed has a primary site of blood loss below the level of the esophagus

3. A lower gastrointestinal bleed has a primary site of blood loss below the ligament of Treitz
4. An upper gastrointestinal bleed has a primary site of blood loss above the level of the esophagus

A. 1, 2, and 3 are correct
B. 1 and 3 are correct
C. 2 and 4 are correct
D. Only 4 is correct
E. All are correct

20. For an alcoholic patient with an acute upper gastrointestinal bleed, the hospital procedure for determining the origin of the bleed is

A. CT scan
B. Endoscopy
C. Ultrasound
D. Exploratory surgery

21. Acute hospital management of bleeding esophageal varices includes
1. Insertion of a Sengstaken-Blakemore tube
2. Direct injection of dopamine into the varix
3. Infusion of vasopressin (Pitressin)
4. Performance of a tracheostomy

A. 1, 2, and 3 are correct
B. 1 and 3 are correct
C. 2 and 4 are correct
D. Only 4 is correct
E. All are correct

Discussion

Your patient's clinical condition represents, in terms of severity, the extreme end of the clinical spectrum seen with gastrointestinal hemorrhage. The marked hypotension, tachycardia, pallor, and obtunded mental state are all indicative of a shock state. The finding of orthostatic changes suggests an approximate 20% acute reduction in intravascular volume. The source of blood loss can be deduced from several factors. The passage of tarry-black, foul-smelling stools reported by your patient is known as melena, and results from blood in the upper gastrointestinal tract that has interacted with gastric and upper intestinal secretions. Along with his history of alcohol abuse, the finding of melena strongly points to the gastrointestinal tract as the site of your patient's blood loss. This conclusion is further supported by the frank hematemesis (vomiting of blood) during transport.

For purposes of localization and treatment, *gastrointestinal hemorrhage* is often classified as either an *upper gastrointestinal bleed* or a *lower gastrointestinal bleed*. The anatomical area of demarcation used for this classification is a structure known as the ligament of Treitz, a fibromuscular band of tissue located around the distal portion of the duodenum. Hemorrhages due to gastritis, esophagitis, peptic ulcer disease, and esophageal varices all originate above the ligament of Treitz and hence are grouped together as upper gastrointestinal bleeds (Figure 5–2).

Gastritis and *esophagitis* are conditions characterized by superficial erosion of the epithelial tissues at the level of the stomach and the esophagus respectively. *Peptic ulcer disease,* commonly called "ulcer" by the lay public, usually involves an ulcerative lesion either in the stomach itself or in the proximal part of the small intestine (duodenum). *Esophageal varices* represent a potentially catastrophic complication most commonly seen in patients with chronic alcoholism and associated liver disease. Engorgement of the veins in the lower esophagus, due to abnormally shunted blood secondary to liver injury, results in the so-called esophageal varices (Figure 5–3). The significance of this condition is that rupture of esophageal varices can result in massive life-threatening upper gastrointestinal hemorrhage.

Hemorrhages due to anorectal tears, colonic polyps, tumors, diverticula, and hemorrhoids originate below the ligament of Treitz and hence are grouped together as lower gastrointestinal bleeds. These sources of hemorrhage are less common as acute life-threatening causes of bleeding and are not strongly associated with a history of alcohol abuse. Your patient's history of chronic alcoholism, the report of

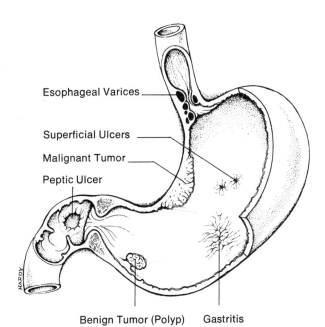

FIGURE 5–2. Common sites and causes of massive upper gastrointestinal bleeding. (Cosgriff JH Jr, Anderson DL: The Practice of Emergency Care, 2nd ed, p 415. Philadelphia, JB Lippincott, 1984)

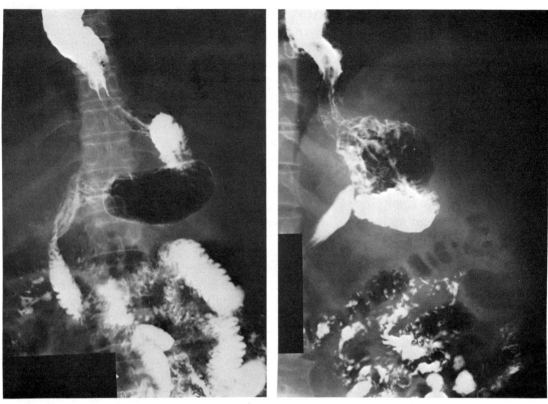

FIGURE 5-3. Esophageal varices. Such varices usually result from portal hypertension. (Cosgriff JH Jr, Anderson DL: The Practice of Emergency Care, 2nd ed, p 416. Philadelphia, JB Lippincott, 1984)

melena over the past several days, and the frank hematemesis all point to a hypovolemic state secondary to an upper gastrointestinal bleed.

Field treatment calls for immediately correcting the patient's hypovolemic shock state. Since a patent airway and spontaneous respirations are present, respiratory management consists of administering supplemental oxygen. Following basic life support measures such as monitoring vital signs, placing the patient in shock position, and oropharyngeal suctioning of blood and vomitus, begin cardiac monitoring. As expected, your patient shows a compensatory sinus tachycardia that requires no specific medical management.

Treatment of the hypovolemia centers around intravascular fluid replacement and use of an external binder device such as military antishock trousers (MAST). Fluid replacement should entail establishing at least one and preferably two large-bore (14 or 16 gauge catheter) intravenous (IV) lines with a "macro" drip administration set. If feasible, draw baseline blood samples both for a rapid field determination of blood glucose levels and for transport to the hospital. The fluid of choice should be either a crystalloid or a colloid, depending upon protocol and experience. The former includes solutions such as normal saline and lactated Ringer's, while the latter includes human plasma protein fraction (Plasmanate), dextran, and albumin. Both colloid solutions and high-salt-containing crystalloid solutions are more effective in acutely expanding intravascular volume than solutions which are predominantly dextrose (D5/W, D5/half normal saline).

Because your patient also shows an altered mental state (which may or may not be related to his gastrointestinal bleed), it is probably wise to administer medications such as thiamine, D50, and naloxone. Thiamine is often administered either IV slow push or IM at a dose between 10 to 100 mg. Next, administer D50 (50 ml of a 50% solution) to correct any underlying hypoglycemia. Lastly, administer naloxone, 0.4 to 0.8 mg as an IV bolus, if the patient has ingested an opiate derivative, such as codeine, pentazocine, Dilaudid, meperidine, or morphine sulfate. Pressor agents such as dopamine and norepinephrine are not called for, since these are best reserved for patients who fail to show improvement following adequate fluid replacement and use of MAST. Further treatment should include frequent monitoring of vital signs during transport.

The initial hospital treatment of a patient such as yours would include continued fluid replacement and transfusion of blood and possibly blood products in order to stabilize his condition. Next, determining the site of the bleed is crucial,

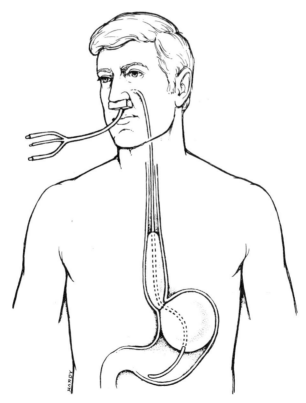

FIGURE 5–4. Sengstaken-Blakemore tube in place. (Cosgriff JH Jr, Anderson DL: The Practice of Emergency Care, 2nd ed, p 418. Philadelphia, JB Lippincott, 1984)

especially when the patient is an alcoholic. Treatment of esophageal variceal bleeding, which is common in alcoholics, differs from treatment of upper gastrointestinal bleeding due to other causes. Localization calls for use of a fiberoptic device to visualize the inside of the gastrointestinal tract, a technique known as *endoscopy*. If esophageal varices are found, as was the case in this patient, one of several treatment options available is the insertion of a Sengstaken-Blakemore tube: a thin, rubber, tubelike device with a balloon which, upon inflation, acts to tampon the engorged bleeding varices (Figure 5-4). Further treatment will vary and may range from continued blood transfusions to surgical intervention.

Field Diagnosis

- Hypovolemic shock
- Upper gastrointestinal bleed
- Altered mental state

Hospital Diagnosis

- Upper gastrointestinal bleed secondary to esophageal varices
- Hypovolemic shock
- Chronic alcoholic liver disease

Patient Follow-Up

Endoscopy confirmed the presence of bleeding esophageal varices. A Sengstaken-Blakemore tube was inserted and blood transfusions continued. Two to three hours later, following transfer to the intensive care unit, and eight hours after arriving in the emergency room, your patient experienced a rebleed that did not respond to aggressive medical management. Shortly thereafter your patient died.

Answers

1. A

    American Academy of Orthopaedic Surgeons: Emergency Care and Transportation of the Sick and Injured, 4th ed, p 132. Menasha, WI, George Banta Co, 1987

    Taber's Cyclopedic Medical Dictionary, 14th ed, sv "melena"

2. A

    Baldwin L, Pierce R: Mobile Intensive Care: A Problem-Oriented Approach, pp 248–250. St Louis, CV Mosby, 1978

    Hart FD (ed): French's Index of Differential Diagnosis, 12th ed, pp 548–549. Littleton, MA, John Wright & Sons, 1985

3. B

    American Academy of Orthopaedic Surgeons: Emergency Care and Transportation of the Sick and Injured, 4th ed, pp 365–367. Menasha, WI, George Banta Co, 1987

    Schuckit MA: Alcoholism and drug dependency. In Braunwald E, Isselbacher KJ, Petersdorf RG (eds): Harrison's Principles of Internal Medicine, 11th ed. New York, McGraw-Hill, 1987

4. D

    Manning RT, Delp MH: Major's Physical Diagnosis, 9th ed, pp 346–348. Philadelphia, WB Saunders, 1981

Schuckit MA: Alcoholism and drug dependency. In Braunwald E, Isselbacher KJ, Petersdorf RG (eds): Harrison's Principles of Internal Medicine, 11th ed. New York, McGraw-Hill, 1987

5. D

Baldwin L, Pierce R: Mobile Intensive Care: A Problem-Oriented Approach, p 261. St Louis, CV Mosby, 1978

6. B

Baldwin L, Pierce R: Mobile Intensive Care: A Problem-Oriented Approach, pp 248–250. St Louis, CV Mosby, 1978

7. C

Braunwald E: Edema. In Braunwald E, Isselbacher KJ, Petersdorf RG (eds): Harrison's Principles of Internal Medicine, 11th ed. New York, McGraw-Hill, 1987

8. A

Manning RT, Delp MH: Major's Physical Diagnosis. 9th ed, p 259. Philadelphia, WB Saunders, 1981
Hart FD (ed): French's Index of Differential Diagnosis, 12th ed, pp 108–112. Littleton, MA, John Wright & Sons, 1985

9. C

American Academy of Orthopaedic Surgeons: Emergency Care and Transportation of the Sick and Injured, 4th ed, p 271. Menasha, WI, George Banta Co, 1987

10. D

Andreoli TE, Carpenter CCJ, Plum F (eds): Cecil's Essentials of Medicine, pp 264–265. Philadelphia, WB Saunders, 1986
Isselbacher KJ, Richter JM: Hematemesis, melena, and hematochezia. In Braunwald E, Isselbacher KJ, Petersdorf RG (eds): Harrison's Principles of Internal Medicine, 11th ed. New York, McGraw-Hill, 1987

11. B

Peterson WL: Gastrointestinal bleeding. In Sleisenger MH, Fordtran JS (eds): Gastrointestinal Disease: Pathophysiology, Diagnosis, and Management. Philadelphia, WB Saunders, 1983
Andreoli TE, Carpenter CCJ, Plum F (eds): Cecil's Essentials of Medicine, pp 263–265. Philadelphia, WB Saunders, 1986

12. B

Walraven G, Harding J, LeBlanc KM et al: Manual of Advanced Prehospital Care, pp 134–135. Bowie, MD, Robert J Brady Co, 1978
Baldwin L, Pierce R: Mobile Intensive Care: A Problem-Oriented Approach, p 261. St Louis, CV Mosby, 1978

13. A

Caroline NL: Ambulance Calls, pp 65–66. Boston, Little, Brown and Co, 1980
Medical Advisory Committee: MAC Paramedic Treatment Protocols. New York, New York City Emergency Medical Services, 1987

14. A

Butman AM, Reinberg SE et al (eds): Advanced Skills in Emergency Care, pp 160–161. Connecticut, Education Direction, 1982

15. C

Butman AM, Reinberg SE et al (eds): Advanced Skills in Emergency Care, pp 160–161. Connecticut, Education Direction, 1982

16. D

Isselbacher KJ, Podolsky DK: Cirrhosis. In Braunwald E, Isselbacher KJ, Petersdorf RG (eds): Harrison's Principles of Internal Medicine, 11th ed. New York, McGraw-Hill, 1987

17. D

Huff J, Doernbach DP, White RD: ECG Workout: Exercises In Arrhythmia Interpretation, pp 11, 213 (strip 1.19). Philadelphia, JB Lippincott, 1985

18. B

DeGowin RL: DeGowin & DeGowin's Bedside Diagnostic Examination, 5th ed, pp 479–480. New York, Macmillan, 1987
American Academy of Orthopaedic Surgeons: Emergency Care and Transportation of the Sick and Injured, 4th ed, pp 348–349. Menasha, WI, George Banta Co, 1987

19. B

Andreoli TE, Carpenter CCJ, Plum F (eds): Cecil's Essentials of Medicine, pp 263–267. Philadelphia, WB Saunders, 1986

20. B

Andreoli TE, Carpenter CCJ, Plum F (eds): Cecil's Essentials of Medicine, pp 263–267. Philadelphia, WB Saunders, 1986

21. B

Peterson WL: Gastrointestinal bleeding. In Sleisenger MH, Fordtran JS (eds): Gastrointestinal Disease: Pathophysiology, Diagnosis, and Management. Philadelphia, WB Saunders, 1983

Selected Reading

Eastwood GL: Upper GI bleeding: differential diagnosis and management (Part 2). Hosp Med 23:44, 1987

Schuckit MA: Alcoholism and drug dependency. In Braunwald E, Isselbacher KJ, Petersdorf RG (eds): Harrison's Principles of Internal Medicine, 11th ed, New York, McGraw-Hill, 1987

Isselbacher KJ, Richter JM: Hematemesis, melena, and hematochezia. In Braunwald E, Isselbacher KJ, Petersdorf RG (eds): Harrison's Principles of Internal Medicine, 11th ed, New York, McGraw-Hill, 1987

6

Chest Pain and Palpitations in a Middle-Aged Man

You and your partner receive a call concerning a "sick male". Upon arrival you find your patient seated in the living room of a small single family house. He has some difficulty relating a story, but his wife reports that he suffered severe chest pain with sweating, lasting approximately thirty minutes. In addition, she tells you that he appeared very pale and vomited several times. She had wanted to call the ambulance, but he insisted that it was just indigestion. Although the pain abated, the patient continued to suffer profuse sweating, nausea, and lightheadedness, along with palpitations. At this point, his wife insisted on calling EMS.

Your patient is a 58-year-old man weighing approximately 160 pounds. Questioning reveals that he is presently experiencing some shortness of breath. His medical history is remarkable for hypertension of many years' duration, treated with clonidine 0.1 mg po bid, which the patient admits he did not take today. He also informs you that he had an inguinal hernia repair three years ago. No history of angina or myocardial infarction is elicited. The patient's father died at age 56 of a heart attack and his younger brother suffers from angina. Reluctantly, he admits to smoking two packs of cigarettes a day ever since he was a teenager and to being a social drinker. He reports no medication allergies and indicates that he has worked in construction for the past 35 years.

Initial vital signs on arrival are BP (right arm, supine) 80 by palpation, pulse 140 and regular with beat-to-beat variation in intensity, respiration 16 and regular, and temperature cool to touch. Physical examination reveals an apprehensive man in mild respiratory distress. Head and neck examination is normal and reveals a patent airway. Thoracic examination shows good symmetrical respiratory excursion with no use of accessory muscles. Auscultation of the lung fields reveals minimal bibasilar rales and otherwise good air exchange. The point of maximal impulse (PMI) is weakly palpable and located in the fifth intercostal space. Heart sounds are normal S_1S_2, although somewhat diminished in intensity. With the patient inclined at a 45-degree angle no jugular venous distension (JVD) is apparent and no hepatojugular reflux (HJR) is elicited. No peripheral edema is noted. Capillary refill is delayed and the skin is cold and clammy. The abdomen is nontender and soft, and no masses are palpated. The remainder of the examination is deferred at this time. Repeat vital signs show BP (right arm, supine) 82 by

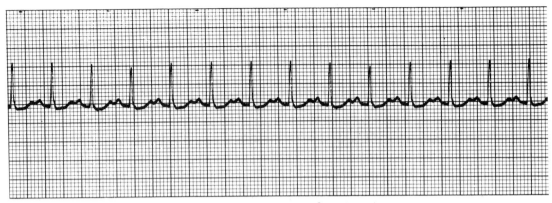

FIGURE 6-1. Lead II EKG recorded prior to initiation of treatment.

palpation, pulse 136 regular and weak, respiration 22 and regular, and temperature cool to touch.

Medical control is contacted, cardiac monitoring is initiated (Figure 6-1), and appropriate field treatment is instituted. With an estimated arrival fifteen minutes later, you begin transport. Ten minutes into transport your cardiac monitor shows the rhythm depicted in Figure 6-2. You quickly consult with medical control and a decision is made to administer a specific medication. During the remainder of transport, the patient's vital signs are BP (right arm, supine) 60 by palpation, pulse 130 irregular and weak, and respiration 28 and regular.

Upon his arrival at the emergency room, a full 12 lead EKG is recorded. The patient's blood is drawn and sent for chemical analysis, an arterial blood gas (ABG) measurement is obtained, cardiac monitoring is continued, and additional medications are administered while the patient is prepared for further procedures.

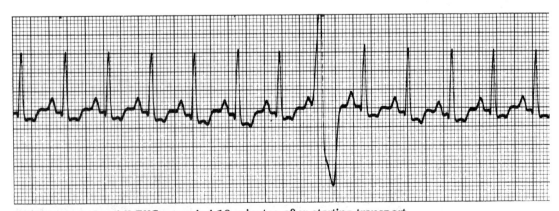

FIGURE 6-2. Lead II EKG recorded 10 minutes after starting transport.

Questions

Read each question carefully, keeping in mind the context of the case under discussion. Select the best answer from the choices presented.

1. Which of the following points in your patient's medical history is not correctly documented under the part of the medical history known as the "history of the present illness"?
   A. Profuse sweating
   B. Palpitations
   C. Regular use of clonidine
   D. Chest pain

2. Your patient claims he is presently being treated with clonidine 0.1 mg po bid. This means that he is taking 0.1 mg of his medication
   A. Once a day orally
   B. Twice a day intravenously
   C. Once a day subcutaneously
   D. Twice a day orally

3. Points in your patient's medical history that are considered risk factors for the development of coronary artery disease include
   A. Smoking and a family history of heart disease
   B. Hypertension and recent travel
   C. Smoking and use of the medication clonidine
   D. Family history of heart disease and occupation as a construction worker

4. Your patient's chest pain and the associated diaphoresis, dyspnea, nausea, and palpitations are most suggestive of which of the following?
   A. Cardiac tamponade
   B. Pulmonary embolism
   C. Peptic ulcer disease
   D. Acute myocardial infarction

5. Shock can best be defined as a physiological state in which there is a(n)
   A. Blood pressure less than 90 mm Hg and a pulse rate of greater than 100 beats per minute
   B. Inadequate perfusion to vital body organs and tissues
   C. Inadequate intravascular volume
   D. Decreased amount of oxygen in the blood

6. Your patient's initial vital signs indicate
   A. Tachycardia and hypertension
   B. Hypotension and tachypnea
   C. Tachycardia and hypotension
   D. Hypotension and apnea

7. The best explanation for the finding of bibasilar rales in your patient is
   A. Decreased right ventricular output leading to increased congestion in the systemic vascular circuit
   B. Decreased left ventricular output leading to increased congestion in the pulmonary vascular circuit
   C. Increased left ventricular output leading to increased congestion in the pulmonary vascular circuit
   D. Increased left ventricular output leading to decreased pulmonary vascular congestion

8. The S_1 component of normal heart sounds reflects
   A. Opening of the mitral valve and opening of the tricuspid valve
   B. Closing of the aortic valve and closing of the pulmonic valve
   C. Opening of the aortic valve and closing of the pulmonic valve
   D. Closing of the mitral valve and closing of the tricuspid valve

9. Field treatment of your patient is best based on a field diagnosis of
   A. Cor pulmonale
   B. Cardiogenic shock
   C. Acute pulmonary edema
   D. Congestive heart failure

10. Basic life support of your patient should include all of the following procedures except
    A. Administration of an enriched supplemental oxygen mixture
    B. Monitoring of vital signs
    C. Application of venous constricting bands (VCBs)
    D. Placement in a supine or semi-sitting position

11. Advanced life support treatment of your patient should include which of the following procedures?
    A. Establishment of a peripheral intravenous line, use of vasopressor agents, and constant cardiac monitoring
    B. Immediate endotracheal intubation, cardiac monitoring, and use of vasopressor agents
    C. Establishment of a peripheral intravenous line, use of analgesic medications (*i.e.*, morphine sulfate), and constant cardiac monitoring

12. Inotropic agents that may help to stabilize your patient's blood pressure include
    A. Nitroglycerin and morphine sulfate
    B. Isoproterenol and calcium chloride
    C. Dobutamine and dopamine
    D. Lidocaine and norepinephrine

13. Following your initial treatment your patient shows no clinical improvement. The next measure you should consider is

A. A fluid challenge
B. Synchronized cardioversion
C. Application of VCBs
D. Nonsynchronized defibrillation

14. The initial EKG depicted in Figure 6-1 is best classified as
    A. Sinus bradycardia
    B. Normal sinus rhythm
    C. Ventricular tachycardia
    D. Sinus tachycardia

15. Which of the following approaches is best for treating the rhythm seen in Figure 6-1?
    A. Administration of morphine sulfate
    B. Synchronized cardioversion
    C. Administration of atropine
    D. No direct treatment (correct underlying problem)

16. Your patient's cardiac rhythm monitored during transport and shown in Figure 6-2 is best classified as
    A. Sinus tachycardia with premature atrial contractions
    B. Normal sinus rhythm with aberrant conduction
    C. Sinus tachycardia with premature ventricular contractions
    D. Normal sinus rhythm with a premature junctional contraction

17. After consulting with medical control, the medication you are most likely to administer is
    A. Lidocaine
    B. Atropine
    C. Epinephrine
    D. Bretylium tosylate

18. Cardiogenic shock is a clinical state manifested by
    A. Severe cardiac arrhythmias leading to inadequate cardiac output
    B. Severe congestive heart failure
    C. Inadequate intravascular volume leading to decreased venous return and decreased cardiac output
    D. Extensive myocardial damage resulting in pump failure with inadequate cardiac output and organ perfusion

19. Cardiogenic shock is usually associated with a mortality rate of approximately
    A. 1%
    B. 30%
    C. 50%
    D. 80%

20. Which of the following statements concerning the medication dopamine is incorrect?
   A. At doses of 1 and 2 ug/kg/min it has primarily a dopamine receptor stimulating action
   B. At doses above 10 ug/kg/min it has primarily an α-receptor stimulating action
   C. At doses between 2 and 10 ug/kg/min it has a β-receptor stimulating action
   D. At doses of 0.5 to 1.0 ug/kg/min it has primarily an α-receptor stimulating action

Discussion

Your patient is in a shocklike state, with symptoms including chest pain, dyspnea, hypotension, tachycardia, and some pulmonary congestion. These findings, in conjunction with his clinical history, suggest a field diagnosis of cardiogenic shock.

Cardiogenic shock is usually the result of extensive damage to the left ventricular myocardium, resulting in the inability of the heart to maintain forward cardiac output. This "pump failure" results in inadequate perfusion of the vital body organs and tissues. The effects of this inadequate perfusion are apparent in your patient (Figure 6-3). Lightheadedness results from decreased cerebral perfusion. Attempts to shunt blood to vital body organs (heart, brain, liver) cause peripheral vasoconstriction and explain the patient's cool, pale skin. His hypotensive state is due to the inability of the left ventricle to pump blood forward into the systemic system and thereby maintain blood pressure. Furthermore, because blood cannot be pumped forward out of the left ventricle, it backs up into the pulmonary vascular circuit and causes pulmonary congestion in the form of bibasilar rales.

Cardiogenic shock commonly results from massive myocardial infarction. In this case, the patient's medical history reveals multiple risk factors that predispose him to coronary artery disease. These factors include hypertension, smoking, and a family history of cardiovascular disease. The 30-minute episode of chest pain and diaphoresis reported by the patient's wife should suggest the strong possibility that the patient suffered an acute myocardial infarction (AMI). Massive damage to the heart muscle probably resulted in the symptom complex known as cardiogenic shock. As a rule, this form of shock is extremely serious because of its high mortality rate (approximately 80%). Aggressive measures must therefore be taken to rectify your patient's hemodynamic status (Table 6-1).

Initial treatment should include administering an enriched supplemental oxygen mixture. Although not called for in this case, in cases of cardiogenic shock where there is serious respiratory insufficiency, intubation may be necessary. Position the patient for maximum perfusion of the vital organs. Place him in a supine position to maximize cerebral perfusion; modify to a semi-sitting position if the patient experiences increased difficulty breathing.

Cardiac monitoring to detect and correct any life-threatening arrhythmias should be instituted early. The patient's initial cardiac rhythm (sinus tachycardia) is typical; his body must compensate for low blood pressure. The later EKG rhythm

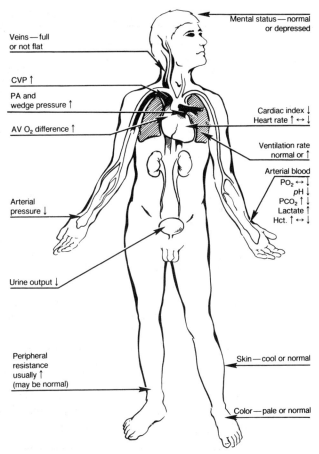

FIGURE 6-3. Cardiogenic shock. Clinical and physiological effects. (Hardy JD [ed]: Hardy's Textbook of Surgery, 2nd ed, p 33. Philadelphia, JB Lippincott, 1988)

showing sinus tachycardia with premature ventricular contractions may, depending on local protocols, require treatment with an anti-arrhythmic agent such as lidocaine. Establishing a peripheral intravenous (IV) line is vital because fluid and medication routes are mandatory. Due to the patient's marked hypotension, agents such as morphine sulfate and verapamil should be avoided because they may lead to further hypotension and cardiac insufficiency, respectively. In such cases it is often prudent to attempt a fluid challenge, either separately or in conjunction with the use of pressor agents. A fluid challenge involves rapidly administering a set amount of IV fluids over a short period of time, while monitoring mental status and vital signs. In cases of cardiogenic shock a fluid challenge may act either beneficially to increase forward cardiac output, or harmfully to increase pulmonary congestion; therefore, it must be undertaken with extreme care. If pulmonary congestion occurs, a diuretic such as furosemide (Lasix) may be required to relieve impending or frank pulmonary edema. Using vasopressor agents to treat cardio-

TABLE 6-1. Management of Cardiogenic Shock

Treatment Modality	Comments
Administer supplemental enriched oxygen	
Establish IV line with D5/W	Consider fluid challenge
Initiate cardiac monitoring	Watch for development of malignant ventricular arrhythmias
Obtain baseline blood samples for transport to hospital	
Reevaluate clinical status and vital signs at frequent intervals	Be especially alert for development of pulmonary edema, cardiac arrhythmias, and hypotension

Medication Options	Comments
Dopamine, 2-5 ug/kg/min, IV infusion titrated till adequate blood pressure is obtained	Use when marked hypotension and evidence of inadequate tissue perfusion are present
or	
Dobutamine, 2.5-5 ug/kg/min, IV infusion, titrated till adequate blood pressure is obtained or maximum dose of 10 ug/kg/min is administered	
Lidocaine, 1 mg/kg IV bolus; additional 0.5 mg/kg boluses every 10 min if required, to a maximum dose of 3 mg/kg; follow with a 2-4 mg/min IV infusion	Use when clinically significant ventricular ectopy is present

genic shock increases cardiac output and peripheral vascular resistance, both of which help raise the patient's systemic arterial blood pressure. Commonly used pressor agents include dobutamine and dopamine.

> **Field Diagnosis**
> - Acute myocardial infarction
> - Cardiogenic shock
>
> **Hospital Diagnosis**
> - Extensive anterior wall myocardial infarction
> - Cardiogenic shock

Patient Follow-Up

Your patient was admitted to the coronary care unit. Despite aggressive treatment with vasopressors he remained hypotensive and suffered decreased cardiac output. On his second day in the hospital he went into cardiopulmonary arrest; despite aggressive measures, he could not be resuscitated.

Answers

1. **C**
   Delp MH, Manning RT: Major's Physical Diagnosis, 9th ed, pp 15–26. Philadelphia, WB Saunders, 1981
   DeGowin RL: DeGowin & DeGowin's Bedside Diagnostic Examination, 5th ed, pp 14–36. New York, Macmillan, 1987

2. **D**
   Taber's Cyclopedic Medical Dictionary, 14th ed, sv "bid"

3. **A**
   American Academy of Orthopaedic Surgeons: Emergency Care and Transportation of the Sick and Injured, 4th ed, p 310. Menasha, WI, George Banta Co, 1987
   Grant HD, Murray RH Jr, Bergeron JD: Emergency Care, 4th ed, p 345. Bowie, MD, Robert J Brady Co, 1986

4. **D**
   American Academy of Orthopaedic Surgeons: Emergency Care and Transportation of the Sick and Injured, 4th ed, pp 312–316. Menasha, WI, George Banta Co, 1987
   Goldberger E, Wheat MW Jr: Treatment of Cardiac Emergencies, 3rd ed, pp 140–165. St Louis, CV Mosby, 1982

5. **B**
   American Academy of Orthopaedic Surgeons: Emergency Care and Transportation of the Sick and Injured, 4th ed, p 134. Menasha, WI, George Banta Co, 1987
   Guyton AC: Textbook of Medical Physiology, 6th ed, pp 332–343. Philadelphia, WB Saunders, 1981

6. **C**
   American Academy of Orthopaedic Surgeons: Emergency Care and Transportation of the Sick and Injured, 4th ed, pp 605, 622. Menasha, WI, George Banta Co, 1987

7. **B**
   Goldberger E, Wheat MW Jr: Treatment of Cardiac Emergencies, 3rd ed, p 40. St Louis, CV Mosby, 1982
   American Academy of Orthopaedic Surgeons: Emergency Care and Transportation of the Sick and Injured, 4th ed, p 314. Menasha, WI, George Banta Co, 1987

8. **D**
   DeGowin RL: DeGowin & DeGowin's Bedside Diagnostic Examination, 5th ed, p 365. New York, Macmillan, 1987
   Andreoli TE, Carpenter CCJ, Plum F (eds): Cecil's Essentials of Medicine, pp 17–18. Philadelphia, WB Saunders, 1986

9. **B**
   Huszar RJ: Emergency Cardiac Care, pp 42–43. Bowie, MD, Robert J Brady Co, 1974
   McIntyre KM, Lewis AJ (eds): Textbook of Advanced Cardiac Life Support, pp III-6–III-8. American Heart Association, 1981
   Goldberger E, Wheat MW Jr: Treatment of Cardiac Emergencies, 3rd ed, pp 38–58. St Louis, CV Mosby, 1982

10. **C**
    Goldberger E, Wheat MW Jr: Treatment of Cardiac Emergencies, 3rd ed, pp 45–52. St Louis, CV Mosby, 1982

11. **A**
    Goldberger E, Wheat MW Jr: Treatment of Cardiac Emergencies, 3rd ed, pp 45–52. St Louis, CV Mosby, 1982
    Fox KAA: Coronary heart disease. In Orland MJ, Saltman RJ (eds): Manual of Medical Therapeutics, 25th ed, p 86. Boston, Little, Brown & Co, 1986

12. **C**
    Fox KAA: Coronary heart disease. In Orland MJ, Saltman RJ (eds): Manual of Medical Therapeutics, 25th ed, pp 85, 86. Boston, Little, Brown & Co, 1986
    Auerbach PS, Budassi SA: Cardiac Arrest and CPR, 2nd ed, pp 51–52. Rockville, MD, Aspen Systems, 1983

13. **A**
    Goldberger E, Wheat MW Jr: Treatment of Cardiac Emergencies, 3rd ed, pp 46–48. St Louis, CV Mosby, 1982

14. **D**
    Huff J, Doernbach DP, White RD: ECG Workout: Exercises in Arrhythmia Interpretation, pp 16, 214 (strip 1.33). Philadelphia, JB Lippincott, 1985
    Alpert MA: Cardiac Arrhythmias, pp 8–10. Chicago, Year Book Medical Publishers, 1980

15. **D**

Alpert MA: Cardiac Arrhythmias, pp 8-10. Chicago, Year Book Medical Publishers, 1980

McIntyre KM, Lewis AJ (eds): Textbook of Advanced Cardiac Life Support, p VI-9. American Heart Association, 1981

16. **C**

Huff J, Doernbach DP, White RD: ECG Workout: Exercises in Arrhythmia Interpretation, pp 140, 241 (strip 4.66). Philadelphia, JB Lippincott, 1985

Alpert MA: Cardiac Arrhythmias, pp 17-33. Chicago, Year Book Medical Publishers, 1980

17. **A**

Meador SA, Field JM: Emergency cardiac care: old drugs, new drugs. J Emerg Care Trans 16:22, 1987

American Heart Association: Standards and guidelines for cardiopulmonary resuscitation (CPR) and emergency cardiac care (ECG). JAMA 255:2905, 1986

18. **D**

American Academy of Orthopaedic Surgeons: Emergency Care and Transportation of the Sick and Injured, 4th ed, p 313. Menasha, WI, George Banta Co, 1987

Fox KAA: Coronary heart disease. In Orland MJ, Saltman RJ (eds): Manual of Medical Therapeutics, 25th ed, p 86. Boston, Little, Brown & Co, 1986

19. **D**

Fox KAA: Coronary heart disease. In Orland MJ, Saltman RJ (eds): Manual of Medical Therapeutics, 25th ed, pp 85, 86. Boston, Little, Brown & Co, 1986

20. **D**

McIntyre KM, Lewis AJ (eds): Textbook of Advanced Cardiac Life Support, p IX-3. American Heart Association, 1981

American Heart Association: Standards and guidelines for cardiopulmonary resuscitation (CPR) and emergency cardiac care (ECG). JAMA 255:2905, 1986

Selected Reading

American Heart Association: Standards and guidelines for cardiopulmonary resuscitation (CPR) and emergency cardiac care (ECG). JAMA 255:2905, 1986

Goldberger E, Wheat MW Jr: Treatment of Cardiac Emergencies, 3rd ed, pp 45-52. St Louis, CV Mosby, 1982

Hancock EW: Ischemic heart disease: Acute myocardial infarction. In Rubenstein E, Federman DD (eds): Medicine, pp X-1-X-22. New York, Scientific American, 1987

7

An Unconscious Man with Impending Respiratory Failure

You and your partner are dispatched to aid an "unconscious male." After a short response interval, you pull up in front of a shabby old building and are led inside by the police. In the hallway you find a young man in his late teens lying face up on the floor. He is unconscious and responsive only to deep pain. No signs of external trauma are evident. His vital signs are BP (right arm, supine) 98/68, pulse 54 and regular, and respiration 5 regular and shallow. His pupils are round, equal, and approximately 1 mm in diameter. The oropharynx shows no foreign debris, blood, or vomitus. Lung sounds are decreased bilaterally with a few scattered rhonchi.

Your partner hyperventilates the patient using a bag valve mask, and then intubates him with a size 8 endotracheal tube to improve his poor respiratory status. You attempt to place a peripheral intravenous (IV) line, but after repeated attempts at finding a suitable vein in the forearm are unsuccessful, you elect to place an external jugular line. Following successful intubation and external jugular cannulation, appropriate medications are given and cardiac monitoring is begun (Figure 7–1).

Within 15 seconds of administering the medications, the patient regains consciousness, becomes agitated, and appears able to respond to verbal commands. Despite attempts to restrain him, he continues to show signs of agitation and successfully pulls out the endotracheal tube. Repeat vital signs are now BP (right arm, sitting) 106/78, pulse 64 and regular, and respiration 12 and regular. Pupils are round, equal, and 4 mm in diameter. Further physical assessment is impossible because of your patient's extremely agitated state; a decision is made to commence transport.

Questions

Read each question carefully, keeping in mind the context of the case under discussion. Select the best answer from the choices presented.

1. Which of the following conditions may produce an acutely altered mental state with loss of consciousness?
    1. Insulin shock

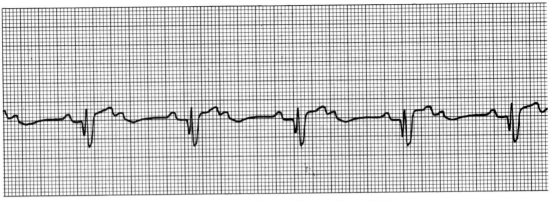

FIGURE 7-1. Lead II EKG recorded shortly after arrival at the scene.

  2. Drug overdose
  3. Cerebrovascular accident
  4. Malignant cardiac arrhythmia (*eg* ventricular fibrillation)

  A. 1, 2, and 3 are correct
  B. 1 and 3 are correct
  C. 2 and 4 are correct
  D. Only 4 is correct
  E. All are correct

2. Symmetrical and markedly constricted pupils may be seen with
   A. Opiate overdose
   B. Spinal lesions
   C. Anticholinergic overdose
   D. Diabetic ketoacidosis

3. Slow and shallow respiration (such as your patient's) often accompanies
   1. Barbiturate overdose
   2. Diabetic ketoacidosis
   3. Opiate overdose
   4. Acetaminophen overdose

   A. 1, 2, and 3 are correct
   B. 1 and 3 are correct
   C. 2 and 4 are correct
   D. Only 4 is correct
   E. All are correct

4. The combination of coma, constricted pupils, and depressed respiration in this patient suggests a field diagnosis of
   A. Pulmonary embolism

B. Cocaine overdose
C. Opiate overdose
D. Diabetic ketoacidosis
E. Acute myocardial infarction

5. The external jugular vein is formed by the union of which of the following pairs of veins?
    A. Posterior facial vein and posterior auricular vein
    B. Internal jugular vein and carotid vein
    C. Subclavian vein and internal jugular vein
    D. Superficial temporal vein and azygous vein

6. When attempting external jugular vein cannulation the patient should be positioned in a supine
    A. Head-down position with the head turned to the side opposite the intended venipuncture site
    B. Head-down position with the head turned towards the side of the intended venipuncture site
    C. Head-up position with the head kept in a midline position
    D. Head-up position with the head turned toward the side of the intended venipuncture site

7. When performing external jugular vein cannulation the cannula should be inserted at a point midway between the
    A. Angle of the jaw and the midclavicular line
    B. Cricothyroid cartilage and the chin
    C. Midclavicular line and the chin
    D. Angle of the jaw and the suprasternal notch

8. The device used for exposing the glottis during endotracheal intubation is known as a
    A. Proctoscope
    B. Magill forceps
    C. Bronchoscope
    D. Laryngoscope

9. The space between the base of the tongue and the epiglottis is known as the
    A. Uvula
    B. Glottic opening
    C. Vallecula
    D. Arytenoid cartilage

10. Appropriate medications for initial administration to this patient include
    1. Naloxone
    2. D50
    3. Thiamine
    4. Valium

A. 1, 2, and 3 are correct
B. 1 and 3 are correct
C. 2 and 4 are correct
D. Only 4 is correct
E. All are correct

11. Your patient's initial cardiac rhythm (Figure 7-1) is best classified as
    A. Paroxysmal atrial tachycardia with variable AV block
    B. Complete third degree AV block
    C. Accelerated idioventricular rhythm
    D. Sinus tachycardia with 2:1 second degree AV block

12. Other notable features of this EKG (Figure 7-1) are
    A. Marked ST segment elevation
    B. Wide QRS complexes
    C. Prolonged QT interval
    D. Grossly abnormal P wave morphology

13. Management of your patient's initial cardiac rhythm (Figure 7-1) should include
    A. Isoproterenol infusion at 30 mg/min
    B. Synchronized dc cardioversion at 50 joules
    C. Lidocaine, 100 mg bolus with a 3 mg/min infusion
    D. None of the above

14. A clinical response to naloxone administration might be expected when intoxication is due to
    1. Heroin
    2. Cocaine
    3. Methadone
    4. Barbiturates

    A. 1, 2, and 3 are correct
    B. 1 and 3 are correct
    C. 2 and 4 are correct
    D. Only 4 is correct
    E. All are correct

15. Naloxone is classified as a(n)
    A. Opiate antagonist
    B. β-adrenergic agonist
    C. Opiate agonist
    D. Calcium channel blocker

16. The purpose of administering D50 to a patient with an altered mental state is to
    A. Provide an increased energy source to the heart muscle

B. Rapidly expand intravascular cerebral volume
C. Correct any underlying hypoglycemia
D. Reverse opiate intoxication

17. The purpose of administering thiamine to a patient with an altered mental state is to
    A. Reverse or prevent alcohol-related neurologic syndromes (*eg* Wernicke-Korsakoff disease)
    B. Reverse symptoms of opiate intoxication (thiamine binds to CNS opiate receptors)
    C. Reverse symptoms of hypoglycemia (thiamine increases blood glucose levels)
    D. Increase cerebral perfusion

18. Pharmacological actions of opiates include
    1. Analgesia
    2. Constipation
    3. Nausea
    4. Respiratory depression

    A. 1, 2, and 3 are correct
    B. 1 and 3 are correct
    C. 2 and 4 are correct
    D. Only 4 is correct
    E. All are correct

19. If during transport to the hospital your patient showed clinical deterioration including lethargy, respiratory depression, and constricted pupils, the best explanation for this would be
    A. Naloxone may cause a syndrome resembling opiate intoxication
    B. The effect of the intoxicating opiate lasts longer than that of the administered naloxone
    C. The effect of naloxone may be counteracted by simultaneously administering thiamine
    D. Naloxone may have an adverse effect upon cerebral perfusion

20. Which of the following represents an incorrect dose and route of administration?
    A. D50, 50 ml of 50% dextrose (25 gm) as an IV bolus
    B. Naloxone, 0.4 mg slow IV bolus
    C. Thiamine, 0.5 mg subcutaneously

Discussion

The causes of unconsciousness and coma are multiple (see "Common Causes of an Altered Mental State"). The specific etiology is often difficult to determine in the

Common Causes of an Altered Mental State

- Cerebrovascular accident
- Meningitis
- Cardiac arrhythmias
- Seizure disorder
- Central nervous system trauma
- Diabetic ketoacidosis
- Insulin shock
- Anoxia
- Hepatic coma
- Uremia
- Septic shock
- Heat stroke
- Drug intoxication
- Structural lesions of the CNS
- Circulatory collapse

field. A systematic approach that attempts to reverse or correct those life-threatening causes of unconsciousness that are amenable to field treatment should be adopted. Initial medical management of this patient, as in all cases, starts with the ABCs, including documenting vital signs (see "Management of Patient with Altered Mental State of Unknown Etiology").

Because your patient shows signs of impending respiratory failure (shallow respirations at 5 per minute), a decision was made to insert an endotracheal tube and assist his ventilation. Insertion of an endotracheal tube is best accomplished by placing the patient in a supine position, with his neck flexed forward and his head extended backward. This puts the head into what has been termed the "sniffing" position and aligns the axes of the mouth, pharynx, and trachea, which facilitates passage of the endotracheal tube. After gathering all the equipment, take the laryngoscope and attached blade in the left hand and an appropriate size endotracheal tube containing a stylet in the right hand. After hyperventilating the patient for several seconds, insert the laryngoscope into his mouth, to the right of the midline. Lift the tongue and displace it towards the left so that the laryngoscope

Management of Patient with an Altered Mental State of Unknown Etiology

Ensure adequate respiratory status.
- Administer oxygen.
- Consider assisted ventilation if required.

Establish intravenous access.
- Use D5/W in cases of "medical emergencies."
- Use NS (or similar fluid) where hypovolemia is suspected.

Initiate cardiac monitoring.
Obtain blood for transport to hospital.
- If possible, perform rapid glucose determination.

Consider medication options.
- Naloxone, 0.4–2.0 mg IV slow push
- Thiamine, 100 mg IV bolus
- Dextrose, 25 gm (50 ml of a 50% solution) IV bolus

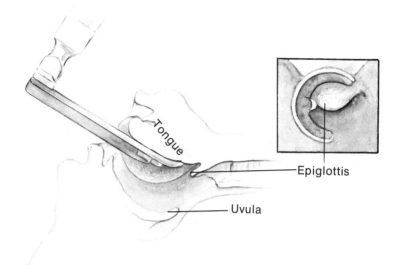

FIGURE 7-2. The laryngoscope is used to visualize structures in the mouth and throat and to facilitate insertion of the endotracheal tube. (Cosgriff JH Jr, Anderson DL: The Practice of Emergency Care, 2nd ed, p 190. Philadelphia, JB Lippincott, 1984)

blade lies in the midline (Figure 7-2). After visualizing the glottic opening, pass the endotracheal tube (held in the right hand) through the mouth and into the trachea (Figure 7-3). Ventilate the patient while someone else auscultates the right and left lung fields and the epigastric area, to confirm that the tube has been placed in the trachea and above the carina. If lung sounds are not heard, or if air passage is auscultated in the epigastric region, then it is likely that the tube lies in the esophagus and not in the trachea. If lung sounds are heard on only one side (most commonly the left), then it is likely that the endotracheal tube was inserted past the carina, and into a mainstem bronchus. The presence of bilaterally equal breath sounds and the absence of any epigastric sounds suggest proper tube placement.

Because medication administration will probably be necessary, and because you could not locate a suitable arm vein, intravenous (IV) access was gained through external jugular cannulation. Placing an IV line in an external jugular vein is often necessary for IV drug abusers, obese patients, and others in whom a suitable arm vein cannot be found. The external jugular vein is formed by the union of the posterior facial vein and the posterior auricular vein. It passes, at the angle of the jaw, from a point behind the ear, over the sternocleidomastoid muscle and under the middle of the clavicle, to join the subclavian vein.

Place the patient in a supine, head-down position (to aid in filling the external jugular veins) and turn the head to the side opposite that intended for venipuncture. After cleaning the skin, locate the vein and direct the cannula toward the ipsilateral shoulder. Insert the cannula at a point midway between the angle of the jaw and the midclavicular line. Finally, tape the line securely in place to prevent inadvertent displacement.

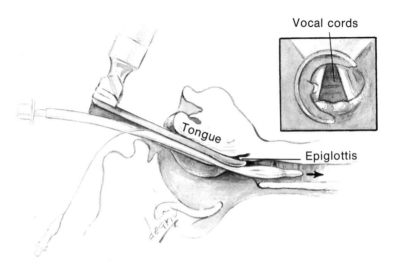

FIGURE 7-3. The endotracheal tube is inserted after the glottic opening is visualized. (Cosgriff JH Jr, Anderson DL: The Practice of Emergency Care, 2nd ed, p 190. Philadelphia, JB Lippincott, 1984)

Cardiac monitoring is an integral part of managing an unconscious patient. This patient's EKG strip reflects a regular rhythm of sinus origin and a ventricular rate of 52. Each QRS complex is preceded by a P wave. There is an atrial rate of 104, however, and not every P wave is followed by a QRS complex. The tracing reveals 2:1 conduction through the AV node, with every other atrial impulse passing through to the ventricles. These findings allow an interpretation of underlying sinus tachycardia with second degree AV block and 2:1 conduction. Treatment of second degree AV block depends on the type and on the patient's clinical state. In cases where an excessively slow ventricular rate is associated with significant hypotension, medications such as atropine or isoproterenol may be indicated, or insertion of a pacemaker may be required. In instances where blood pressure and tissue perfusion appear adequate, such as in this patient, no medical intervention is called for. Treatment consists of continued monitoring in case more malignant arrhythmias develop.

Having successfully intubated your patient and established an intravenous access route, next consider appropriate "medication protocols" for an unconscious individual (Table 7-1). The three medications commonly administered to treat an altered mental state are thiamine, dextrose, and naloxone. Thiamine is administered if alcohol-related neurologic abnormalities such as Wernicke-Korsakoff disease are present. Normally it is administered in a dose ranging from 10 to 100 mg either IV, IM, or a combination of the two. D50 (50% dextrose) is used mainly to correct any underlying hypoglycemic state. A frequently employed dosage is 50 ml of 50% dextrose (25 gm) as an IV bolus. The order in which these two medications are given is at least theoretically important. Because thiamine is used in glucose metabolism, administering large amounts of glucose may, in a patient with mar-

TABLE 7-1. Treatment of Patient with an Acutely Altered Mental State

Medication	Clinical Effects	Administrations
Naloxone	Opiate antagonist; reverses respiratory depression	0.4–2.0 mg slow IV push; may repeat in 3–5 minutes
Thiamine	Prevents or improves Wernicke-Korsakoff syndrome	100 mg, IV bolus
Dextrose	Reverses hypoglycemia	25 gm (50 ml of a 50% solution)

ginal thiamine stores, further deplete available thiamine and precipitate neurologic symptoms. For this reason it is desirable to administer thiamine before dextrose when using both medications.

As the final component of the medication series, administer naloxone to reverse narcotic intoxication (heroin, methadone, morphine sulfate, codeine, etc.). Naloxone is a pure opiate antagonist which competitively blocks ingested opiates by binding to central nervous system opiate receptors. It is highly effective in reversing the marked respiratory depression associated with opiate intoxication. Administration is generally carried out using either the IV, IM, or subcutaneous route; the former is most desirable. The standard adult dose is 0.4 mg to 2 mg slow IV push, repeated at 2 to 5 minute intervals. Clinical improvement usually occurs before a maximum dose (10 mg) can be administered. Recent anecdotal reports suggest that naloxone may have beneficial effects in cases of severe ethanol intoxication, but its widespread use for this purpose is not presently accepted. Jointly administering these three medications will (for the reasons discussed above) often produce rapid clinical improvement in a patient whose altered mental state is linked to opiate intoxication, hypoglycemia, an acute, reversible, alcohol-related neurologic syndrome, or a combination of these conditions. Because these medications produce few or no serious adverse effects, and in some instances may be life saving, they form the core of treatment for the patient with an altered mental state.

Although "medication protocols" such as those outlined above can be safely employed without specific knowledge of the underlying problem, it is often possible to ascertain the etiology of the problem by studying the patient's history and conducting a physical examination. For instance, this patient's triad of symptoms (loss of consciousness, symmetrically constricted pupils, and respiratory depression) is characteristic of opiate intoxication. His rapid clinical improvement following naloxone administration is thus to be expected. It is also common for patients with severe opiate intoxication to become extremely agitated following naloxone administration, as your patient so uncooperatively demonstrated by extubating himself. Remember that because naloxone has a short duration of action compared to the intoxicating opiate, patients may relapse despite initial improvement. For this reason it is always advisable that patients receiving naloxone be transported to a medical facility for further treatment.

> **Field Diagnosis**
> - Ventilatory failure
> - Acutely altered mental state
> - Probable narcotic overdose
>
> **Hospital Diagnosis**
> - Narcotic overdose
> - Second degree heart block, etiology to be determined

Patient Follow-Up

The patient was placed on a continuous naloxone infusion. His blood was drawn for toxicologic and chemical analysis. He remained conscious, and, after 24 hours, was discharged with instructions to return to the clinic for follow-up.

Answers

1. E
   American Academy of Orthopaedic Surgeons: Emergency Care and Transportation of the Sick and Injured, 4th ed, pp 377–381. Menasha, WI, George Banta Co, 1987
   Ropper AH, Martin JB: Coma and other disorders of consciousness. In Braunwald E, Isselbacher KJ, Petersdorf RG (eds): Harrison's Principles of Internal Medicine, 11th ed. New York, McGraw-Hill, 1987

2. A
   American Academy of Orthopaedic Surgeons: Emergency Care and Transportation of the Sick and Injured, 4th ed, p 41. Wisconsin, George Banta Co, 1987
   Baldwin L, Pierce R: Mobile Intensive Care: A Problem-Oriented Approach, p 61. St Louis, CV Mosby, 1978

3. B
   Caroline NL: Ambulance Calls, pp 139–40, 285–87. Boston, Little, Brown & Co, 1980
   Done AK: Of opiates, opiods, and overdoses. Emerg Med 7:242, 1975

4. C
   Hafen BQ, Karren KJ: Prehospital Emergency Care and Crisis Intervention, pp 332–33. Englewood, CO, Morton, 1981
   Baldwin L, Pierce R: Mobile Intensive Care: A Problem-Oriented Approach, pp 199–200. St Louis, CV Mosby, 1978
   Schuckit MA, Segal DS: Opiate drug use. In Braunwald E, Isselbacher KJ, Petersdorf RG (eds): Harrison's Principles of Internal Medicine, 11th ed. New York, McGraw-Hill, 1987

5. A
   McIntyre KM, Lewis AJ (eds): Textbook of Advanced Cardiac Life Support, p XII-4. American Heart Association, 1981

6. A
   McIntyre KM, Lewis AJ (eds): Textbook of Advanced Cardiac Life Support, p XII-5. American Heart Association, 1981

7. A
   McIntyre KM, Lewis AJ (eds): Textbook of Advanced Cardiac Life Support, p XII-4. American Heart Association, 1981
   McIntyre KM, Lewis AJ (eds): Textbook of Advanced Cardiac Life Support, pp IV-4–IV-5. American Heart Association, 1981

8. D
   McIntyre KM, Lewis AJ (eds): Textbook of Advanced Cardiac Life Support, pp IV-4–IV-5. American Heart Association, 1981

9. C

   McIntyre KM, Lewis AJ (eds): Textbook of Advanced Cardiac Life Support, pp IV-4–IV-5. American Heart Association, 1981

10. A

    Andreoli TE, Carpenter CCJ, Plum F (eds): Cecil's Essentials of Medicine, pp 656–657. Philadelphia, WB Saunders, 1986

    Schuckit MA, Segal DS: Opiate drug use. In Braunwald E, Isselbacher KJ, Petersdorf RG (eds): Harrison's Principles of Internal Medicine, 11th ed. New York, McGraw-Hill, 1987

11. D

    Huff J, Doernbach DP, White RD: ECG Workout: Exercises in Arrhythmia Interpretation, pp 79, 226 (strip 3.3). Philadelphia, JB Lippincott, 1985

    Chung EK: Principles of Cardiac Arrhythmias, 3rd ed, pp 63–66. Baltimore, Williams & Wilkins, 1983

12. B

    Huff J, Doernbach DP, White RD: ECG Workout: Exercises in Arrhythmia Interpretation, pp 79, 226 (strip 3.3). Philadelphia, JB Lippincott, 1985

13. D

    American Heart Association: Standards and guidelines for cardiopulmonary resuscitation (CPR) and emergency cardiac care (ECC). JAMA 255:2905, 1986

    Huszar RJ: Emergency Cardiac Care, pp 154–155. Bowie, MD, Robert J Brady Co, 1974

14. B

    Jaffee JH, Martin WR: Opiate analgesics and antagonists. In Gilman AG, Goodman LS, Rall TW (eds): The Pharmacological Basis of Therapeutics, 7th ed. New York, Macmillan, 1985

15. A

    McFeely EJ: Naloxone: a narcotic antagonist. J Emerg Care Trans, 14:70, 1985

    Jaffee JH, Martin WR: Opiate analgesics and antagonists. In Gilman AG, Goodman LS, Rall TW (eds): The Pharmacological Basis of Therapeutics, 7th ed. New York, Macmillan, 1985

16. C

    Baldwin L, Pierce R: Mobile Intensive Care: A Problem-Oriented Approach, pp 169–172. St Louis, CV Mosby, 1978

    American Academy of Orthopaedic Surgeons: Emergency Care and Transportation of the Sick and Injured, 4th ed, pp 335–339. Menasha, WI, George Banta Co, 1987

17. A

    Andreoli TE, Carpenter CCJ, Plum F (eds): Cecil's Essentials of Medicine, pp 676–677. Philadelphia, WB Saunders, 1986

    Marcus R, Coulston AM: Water soluble vitamins. In Gilman AG, Goodman LS, Rall TW (eds): The Pharmacological Basis of Therapeutics, 7th ed, pp 1551–1555. New York, Macmillan, 1985

18. E

    Hafen BQ, Karren KJ: Prehospital Emergency Care and Crisis Intervention, pp 332–333. Englewood, CO, Morton, 1981

    Jaffee JH, Martin WR: Opiate analgesics and antagonists. In Gilman AG, Goodman LS, Rall TW (eds): The Pharmacological Basis of Therapeutics, 7th ed. New York, Macmillan, 1985

19. B

    McFeely EJ: Naloxone: a narcotic antagonist. J Emerg Care Trans, 14:70, 1985

    Jaffee JH, Martin WR: Opiate analgesics and antagonists. In Gilman AG, Goodman LS, Rall TW (eds): The Pharmacological Basis of Therapeutics, 7th ed. New York, Macmillan, 1985

20. C

    Marcus R, Coulston AM: Water soluble vitamins. In Gilman AG, Goodman LS, Rall TW (eds): The Pharmacological Basis of Therapeutics, 7th ed, pp 1551–55. New York, Macmillan, 1985

Selected Reading

Evans LEJ et al: Treatment of drug overdosage with naloxone, a specific antagonist. Lancet 1:452, 1973

Jaffee JH, Martin WR: Opiate analgesics and antagonists. In Gilman AG, Goodman LS,

Rall TW (eds): The Pharmacological Basis of Therapeutics, 7th ed, New York, Macmillan, 1985

Kersh ES: Narcotic overdosage. Hosp Med 10:8, 1974

McFeely EJ: Naloxone: a narcotic antagonist. J Emerg Care Trans, 14:70, 1985

Schuckit MA, Segal DS: Opiate drug use. In Braunwald E, Isselbacher KJ, Petersdorf RG (eds): Harrison's Principles of Internal Medicine, 11th ed, New York, McGraw-Hill, 1987

8

Cough and Fever in a Young Woman

Your ambulance is requested to "respond for" a "sick female." It is five minutes shy of shift change; you glance at your partner, mumble, and copy down the call information. After a 20-minute response interval, you arrive in front of a small two-family house. After securing your vehicle, you gather your equipment and are led inside by a young man in his early 30s. He informs you that his wife, who has been recuperating from abdominal surgery in bed for the past week, started feeling "ill" this evening. While your partner begins taking vital signs, you elicit a history from the patient.

She is a moderately obese woman in her 30s who tells you that she was feeling fine until approximately 1 hour ago, when she started to experience shortness of breath, a nonproductive cough, low-grade fever, and a general sense of fatigue. She denies any chest pain, nausea, vomiting, hemoptysis, hematemesis, chills, palpitations, or recent trauma. Past medical history is remarkable for an appendectomy 1 week ago and a tonsillectomy at age 9. She has no history of angina, myocardial infarction, seizure disorders, cardiac arrhythmia, chronic obstructive pulmonary disease, or recent infection. She reports allergies to penicillin and aspirin, and denies using any prescription medications except for an estrogen-containing contraceptive prescribed by her gynecologist and which she has used for the past 4 years. She has two children and holds a part time clerical job. She admits to "social drinking" and to smoking one pack of cigarettes a day for the past 10 years, but denies recreational drug use. There is no family history of cardiovascular disease, malignancy, diabetes, mental illness, or asthma.

Physical examination findings include the following. Your patient is a 33-year-old woman weighing approximately 180 pounds. She is cooperative and conversant, and appears in mild distress. Vital signs are BP 140/92, pulse 130 and regular, respiration 28 and regular, and temperature 101°F. The head shows no signs of trauma or deformity. The oropharynx is free of foreign debris, gross blood, and vomitus; a small amount of pinkish sputum is noted. The mucous membranes appear cyanotic. The trachea is midline and the neck is without deformity or masses. Jugular venous distension is absent with the patient inclined at a 30-degree angle. Auscultation of the lungs reveals nothing remarkable except for a modestly increased respiratory rate. Auscultation of the heart reveals normal S_1S_2 with a regular rhythm at a rate of approximately 130 beats per minute. The abdomen is

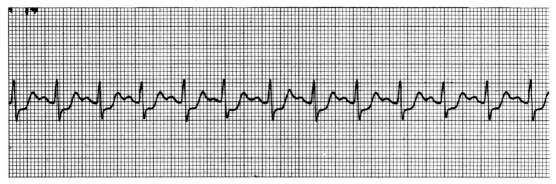

FIGURE 8-1. Lead II EKG recorded shortly after arrival at the scene.

obese and nondistended, and a recent surgical scar in the lower right quadrant is apparent. Bowel sounds are present and normal. The extremities are without deformity, peripheral edema, or ulcerations. No calf pain is elicited by dorsiflexion of either foot or by pressure applied to the posterior calf. Neurologic examination reveals an individual who is alert and oriented to time, place, and person. Sensory and motor function are normal, the cranial nerves appear intact, and no focal abnormalities are noted.

Vital signs repeated 10 minutes after arrival are BP 136/88, pulse 125 and regular, and respiration 28 and regular. You contact medical control, continue cardiac monitoring (Figure 8-1), and administer appropriate treatment during transport. When you arrive at the emergency room with your patient, a chest radiograph and a hemogram are obtained, arterial blood gases are drawn and measured, and a full 12 lead EKG is recorded (Table 8-1 and "Laboratory Values").

Laboratory Values

Chemistries

CBC: WBC 13.6×10^3 cu mm, hemoglobin 14 gm/dl, hematocrit 42%
Serum electrolytes: Na 136 mEq/L, K 3.8 mEq/L, HCO_3 22 mEq/L, and Cl 104 mEq/L
Glucose: 68 mg/dl
Blood urea nitrogen (BUN): 15 mg/dl
Coagulation profile: Normal
Urinalysis: Pending

Radiographs

Chest x-ray: No acute pathology noted

Electrocardiogram

Cardiac monitor: Sinus tachycardia at a rate of 130
12-lead EKG: Sinus tachycardia with nonspecific ST-T changes

TABLE 8-1. Arterial Blood Gas Measurement Performed on Room Air

pH	7.52
Pco	28 mm Hg
Plasma bicarbonate	22 mEq/L
Po	60 mm Hg

Questions

Read each question carefully, keeping in mind the context of the case under discussion. Select the best answer from the choices presented.

1. Your patient's EKG (Figure 8-1) demonstrates which of the following characteristics?
   1. A regular rhythm
   2. Discrete P waves of normal morphology
   3. QRS complexes of normal morphology
   4. Numerous premature atrial contractions

   A. 1, 2, and 3 are correct
   B. 1 and 3 are correct
   C. 2 and 4 are correct
   D. Only 4 is correct
   E. All are correct

2. Your patient's EKG is best classified as
   A. Normal sinus rhythm
   B. Complete third degree AV block
   C. Sinus tachycardia
   D. Atrial fibrillation with rapid ventricular response

3. The arterial blood gas measurement obtained in the hospital shows
   1. Arterial hypoxemia
   2. A low bicarbonate
   3. Arterial hypocapnia
   4. An elevated pH

   A. 1, 2, and 3 are correct
   B. 1 and 3 are correct
   C. 2 and 4 are correct
   D. Only 4 is correct
   E. All are correct

4. The best field diagnosis in this case is
   A. Acute myocardial infarction

B. Spontaneous pneumothorax
C. Pulmonary embolism
D. Septic shock
E. Congestive heart failure

5. Field treatment should include
   1. Placement of an intravenous line
   2. Nitroglycerin, 0.3 mg sublingual
   3. Administration of supplemental oxygen
   4. Furosemide, 40 mg IV bolus

   A. 1, 2, and 3 are correct
   B. 1 and 3 are correct
   C. 2 and 4 are correct
   D. Only 4 is correct
   E. All are correct

Discussion

In this scenario a relatively young woman with no known medical conditions presents with symptoms including an acute onset of dyspnea, fever, and cough. Since this constellation of symptoms suggests a variety of conditions, it is necessary to carefully explore the medical history and the results of the physical examination to clarify the etiology. The patient's medical history includes the following pertinent items: a recent history of abdominal surgery, prolonged bed rest during recovery from surgery, use of an estrogen-containing contraceptive for the past 4 years, a ten-pack-year history of cigarette use, and no known respiratory or cardiovascular disease. Significant physical examination data include obesity, tachycardia (130 beats per minute), tachypnea (28 breaths per minute), pinkish sputum in the oropharynx (possibly representing a small degree of hemoptysis), central cyanosis, and a temperature of 101°F. Also pertinent is the absence of chest pain, abnormal heart sounds, jugular venous distension (JVD), peripheral edema, and pulmonary congestion.

These findings, in addition to the patient's youth, strongly argue against a cardiac etiology such as angina pectoris, acute myocardial infarction (AMI), pericardial tamponade, or congestive heart failure (CHF). Similarly, the patient's youth and moderate smoking history, as well as the absence of diminished breath sounds, hyperresonant lung fields, and marked respiratory distress, make the diagnoses of spontaneous pneumothorax, asthma, bronchitis, or emphysema poor explanations. Pneumonia is a distinct possibility to consider in the prehospital setting, but your patient's chest radiograph, obtained in the hospital, argues against this diagnosis as well. Having eliminated some of the more common causes of dyspnea, fever, and cough, the best diagnosis in this case is pulmonary embolism.

Pulmonary embolism refers to a solid, gaseous, or liquid material that is carried in the blood stream and lodges in the pulmonary vasculature (Table 8-2). Because in virtually all cases the offending agent is a thrombus ("blood clot"), the

TABLE 8-2. Types, Actions, and Causes of Pulmonary Emboli

Type	Action	Causes
Fat embolism	Fat globules enter systemic circulation, occlude pulmonary vasculature, and may produce pulmonary hemorrhage as well as occlusion of blood flow to other organs.	Long bone fractures
Air embolism	A significant amount of air (5–15 ml/kg) enters systemic circulation and lodges in either the right side of the heart or the pulmonary vasculature, thereby obstructing blood flow.	Pneumoperitoneum Accidental IV administration of air
Amniotic fluid embolism	During childbirth amniotic fluid enters the maternal circulation; its solid elements (lanugo, meconium, etc.) lodge in the pulmonary vasculature.	Childbirth
Thromboembolism	Blood clot lodges and occludes the pulmonary vasculature.	Malignancy Obesity Recent abdominal surgery Smoking Estrogen compounds

more specific term pulmonary *thromboembolism* is used; *thrombo-* indicating a blood clot, and *embolism* indicating that the material was carried to the lung from a distant site. Although pulmonary thromboemboli have diverse origins, by far the vast majority arise from thrombi that form in the *deep venous system* of the lower extremities (femoral, iliac, and popliteal veins). Other sites, such as superficial varicose veins (common in older patients) and veins of the calf muscles, are far less common sites of origin. Pulmonary thromboembolism is thus best recognized, diagnosed, treated, and prevented as a complication of deep venous thrombosis (DVT).

Because the presentation of pulmonary thromboembolism is often nonspecific, it is important to recognize both the physiological abnormalities and the clinical conditions that predispose a person to pulmonary embolism. Classically, the pathophysiological abnormalities which place a person at increased risk include stasis, injury or abnormality of the blood vessel wall, and alterations in the coagulation system. These abnormalities are likely to exist in the following situations:

- Venous disease of the lower extremities
- Malignancy
- Postpartum period
- CHF
- Lower extremity fractures
- Recent abdominal surgery
- Prolonged bed rest
- Obesity
- Use of estrogen-containing contraceptives

The possibility of pulmonary thromboembolism should be thoughtfully entertained if one or more of these risk factors exists. At least four pertain to your patient: recent abdominal surgery, prolonged bed rest, obesity, and use of estrogen-containing birth control pills.

The clinical presentation of pulmonary thromboembolism is best understood by first examining its pathophysiological effects on the cardiovascular and respiratory systems. When a thromboembolism lodges in the pulmonary vasculature, it blocks pulmonary arterial blood flow to the alveoli supplied by the occluded vessel. The result is that a portion of the lung contains alveoli that are being ventilated but not perfused (by blood). This unequal distribution of ventilation and perfusion, along with an increased respiratory rate and several other factors, leads to abnormalities in the exchange of carbon dioxide and oxygen. These abnormalities include low arterial oxygen (hypoxemia), low carbon dioxide levels (hypocapnia), and respiratory alkalosis. The effects on the cardiovascular system depend on the size, location, and extent of thromboembolic occlusion. If there is massive occlusion of the main pulmonary artery *(saddle embolus)* then almost complete blockage of pulmonary arterial blood flow may result; collapse and sudden death may follow. In less severe cases, where thromboemboli cause significant, but not complete, obstruction of pulmonary blood flow, pulmonary hypertension and acute right-sided heart failure may result *(acute cor pulmonale)*. Finally, when only minimal to moderate obstruction of pulmonary blood flow occurs, cardiac function may remain essentially intact, with little more than clinically apparent tachycardia and dyspnea resulting.

The clinical presentation of pulmonary thromboembolism is extremely variable for the reasons discussed (see "Clinical Presentation of Pulmonary Thromboembolism"). Perhaps most common is the acute onset of unexplained dyspnea. The patient usually has no history of similar episodes, and no obvious precipitating cause is discernible. Less common are complaints of pleuritic chest pain, hemoptysis, or syncope. The most frequent physical examination finding is the combination of tachypnea, tachycardia, and fever. Other less common, nonspecific findings include scattered rales, an increased intensity of the second heart sound, systolic cardiac murmurs, and various cardiac arrhythmias. The EKG characteristically reflects sinus tachycardia. In sum, unexplained dyspnea accompanied by tachypnea, tachycardia, and fever, in a patient with any of the risk factors listed above, should immediately raise the suspicion of pulmonary thromboembolism.

Your patient's chief complaints, dyspnea and cough, along with the multiple factors that place her at risk of developing pulmonary thromboembolism (obesity, recent surgery, prolonged bed rest, and use of birth control pills), should quickly raise this diagnostic possibility. The physical findings of tachypnea, tachycardia, and fever, in the absence of significant past medical history or other significant findings, also strongly support this diagnosis. Prehospital treatment of this patient, and of pulmonary thromboembolism in general, is largely supportive and aimed at maintaining adequate cardiovascular and pulmonary function (Table 8–3). Monitor vital signs frequently and attend carefully to changes that might foreshadow impending cardiovascular deterioration (hypotension, irregular pulse rate, etc.). Promptly institute cardiac monitoring and watch for the development of malignant arrhythmias. Establish an intravenous line, D5/W, at a keep-vein-open (KVO) rate to provide access in case complications require rapid administration of medica-

Clinical Presentation of Pulmonary Thromboembolism

Chief Complaint

Dyspnea
Cough
Hemoptysis
Pleuritic chest pain

Pertinent Past Medical History

I. Medical History
   A. Congestive heart failure
   B. Malignancy
   C. Lower extremity venous disease
   D. Coagulation defects

II. Surgical History
   A. Recent pelvic surgery
   B. Recent abdominal surgery
   C. Recent fractures

III. Medication History
   A. Use of estrogen-containing contraceptives

IV. Psychosocial History
   A. Obesity
   B. Smoking
   C. Prolonged bed rest (recovering from illness)

Physical Findings

COMMON	LESS COMMON
Tachypnea	Rales
Tachycardia	Abnormal heart sounds
Fever	Systolic cardiac murmurs
	Cardiac arrhythmias

TABLE 8-3. Management of Pulmonary Thromboembolism

Therapeutic Modality	Comment
Monitor vital signs	Watch for hypotension or ineffective ventilatory status
Administer supplemental oxygen	6-8 1/min via face mask or 2-4 1/min via nasal cannula if former is not tolerated
Establish IV line	Peripheral line with D5/W at a KVO rate is sufficient in most cases
Initiate cardiac monitoring	Monitor carefully for development of malignant cardiac arrhythmias; sinus tachycardia is common and in most cases calls for no specific treatment
Transport to medical facility	

tions. Since arterial hypoxemia is common, an enriched supplemental oxygen mixture should be provided. Transport to a medical facility where further treatment can be carried out is mandatory.

Field Diagnosis

- Pulmonary thromboembolism

Hospital Diagnosis

- Pulmonary thromboembolism

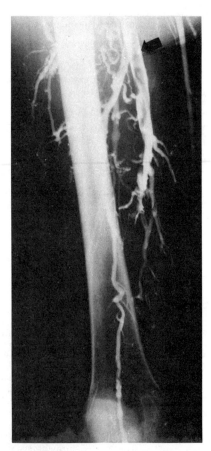

FIGURE 8–2. Contrast venography shows a free-floating thrombus within the femora vein (*arrow*). (Hardy JD (ed): Hardy's Textbook of Surgery, 2nd ed, p 973. Philadelphia, JB Lippincott, 1988)

Patient Follow-Up

Based on the clinical history and laboratory findings, your patient was admitted to the hospital with a diagnosis of pulmonary embolism. A repeat chest radiograph the following day revealed a parenchymal infiltrate and evidence of a pleural effusion. Contrast venography revealed deep venous thrombosis in the lower extremities (Figure 8-2), and ventilation-perfusion scans of the lung confirmed the diagnosis of pulmonary embolism. Anticoagulation was carried out for 10 days, after which the patient was discharged.

Answers

1. A
   Huff J, Doernbach DP, White RD: ECG Workout: Exercises in Arrhythmia Interpretation, pp 26, 216 (strip 1.63). Philadelphia, JB Lippincott, 1985

2. C
   Huff J, Doernbach DP, White RD: ECG Workout: Exercises in Arrhythmia Interpretation, pp 26, 216 (strip 1.63). Philadelphia, JB Lippincott, 1985

3. E
   Shapiro BA, Harrison RA, Walton JR: Clinical Application of Blood Gases, 3rd ed, p 135. Chicago, Year Book Medical Publishers, 1982
   McIntyre KM, Lewis AJ (eds): Textbook of Advanced Cardiac Life Support, pp X-1–X-6. American Heart Association, 1981

4. C
   American Academy of Orthopaedic Surgeons: Emergency Care and Transportation of the Sick and Injured, 4th ed, pp 328–329. Menasha, WI, George Banta Co, 1987
   Moser KM: Pulmonary thromboembolism. In Braunwald E, Isselbacher KJ, Petersdorf RG (eds): Harrison's Principles of Internal Medicine, 11th ed. New York, McGraw-Hill, 1987
   Andreoli TE, Carpenter CCJ, Plum F (eds): Cecil's Essentials of Medicine, pp 152–153. Philadelphia, WB Saunders, 1986

5. B
   American Academy of Orthopaedic Surgeons: Emergency Care and Transportation of the Sick and Injured, 4th ed, p 333. Menasha, WI, George Banta Co, 1987

Selected Reading

Bell WR, Simon TL: Current status of pulmonary thromboembolic disease. Am Heart J 103:239, 1982

Hockberger RS: Pulmonary embolism. In Tintinalli JE, Rothstein RJ, Krome RL (eds): Emergency Medicine: A Comprehensive Study Guide, pp 187–91. New York, McGraw-Hill, 1985

Moser KM: Pulmonary thromboembolism. In Braunwald E, Isselbacher KJ, Petersdorf RG (eds): Harrison's Principles of Internal Medicine, 11th ed. New York, McGraw Hill, 1987

Rosenow EC: Pulmonary embolism. Mayo Clin Proc 56:161, 1981

9

Chest Pain and Dyspnea

Your ambulance is asked to respond to a call involving a middle-aged man with shortness of breath. You arrive and find your patient sitting in bed, profusely diaphoretic and severely tachypneic. His wife informs you that her husband is 53 years old and has a long history of "heart problems." He was hospitalized 1 year ago for a heart attack and has had frequent episodes of exertional chest pain since that time. You learn also that he has had a history of high blood pressure since his early 30s, and that he was recently diagnosed with cirrhosis resulting from years of heavy drinking. His medications include the following: furosemide 40 mg po od, digoxin 0.25 mg po od, methyldopa (Aldomet) 250 mg po bid, KCl 40 mEq po od, multivitamins, diazepam (Valium) 2.5 mg po tid, nitroglycerin tablets, and nitroglycerin paste 1 inch q 6 hours.

Despite his dyspnea, your patient is able to explain that over the past week he has had increasing pressurelike chest pain, frequent bouts of shortness of breath that awaken him from sleep (PND), and a severe cough. He tells you that he now sleeps on three pillows instead of his usual one pillow. He awoke from sleep coughing and extremely short of breath 2 hours ago. Making his way to the toilet, he experienced severe retrosternal chest pain which he describes as "squeezing" and radiating to his jaw. The pain, he reports, decreased in intensity shortly after he took two nitroglycerin tablets. His shortness of breath continued, however, to increase to the point where his wife called for the ambulance. On further questioning, he admits to a history of penicillin allergy.

Your initial impression is of a debilitated, unkempt man who appears markedly dyspneic and diaphoretic and who is using accessory muscles for respiration. His vital signs are BP (right arm, sitting) 180/110, pulse 80 and irregular, and respiration 36 and regular. The pupils appear round, equal, and reactive to light. Examination of the neck shows marked jugular venous distension (JVD) with a positive hepatojugular reflux (HJR). Upon auscultation, lung fields evidence bilateral rales two thirds of the way up. The apical pulse (PMI) is palpated at the seventh intercostal space in the midaxillary line. Heart sounds, though masked by diffuse rales, are present. A loud murmur and a gallop are appreciated. Bowel sounds are present. Extremities reveal 3 plus pitting edema bilaterally. No cyanosis or clubbing is noted. Capillary refill is diminished and distal pulses, although present, are weak. Neurologic examination indicates an alert and oriented individual with no gross abnormalities. The initial EKG is presented in Figure 9–1.

You establish an intravenous (IV) line, monitor vital signs, and administer

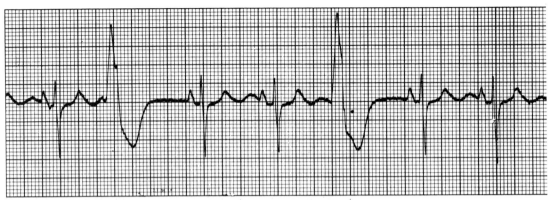

FIGURE 9-1. Lead II EKG recorded shortly after arrival at the scene.

appropriate treatment. Your patient's symptoms decrease somewhat following treatment, and transport proceeds to the nearest hospital. No problems are encountered en route.

Questions

Read each question carefully, keeping in mind the context of the case under discussion. Select the best answer from the choices presented.

1. Acute pulmonary edema of cardiac etiology is due to
   A. Impaired ability of the left side of the heart to pump blood into the systemic circulation, with subsequent backup and increased pressure in the pulmonary circulation
   B. Impaired ability of the left side of the heart to pump blood into the pulmonary circuit, with subsequent backup and increased pressure in the systemic circulation
   C. A toxic effect resulting in an increase in pulmonary alveolar-capillary permeability
   D. An increase in the pressure in the pulmonary circuit, resulting from an increased pumping ability of the right side of the heart

2. Your patient's initial EKG (Figure 9-1) is best classified as
   A. Sinus tachycardia with frequent premature atrial contractions
   B. Ventricular fibrillation
   C. Second degree AV block
   D. Sinus rhythm with frequent premature ventricular contractions

3. An intravenous line
   A. Should be established with normal saline and at a maximum drip rate

B. Is contraindicated in this patient since fluid load must be restricted
C. Should be started with D5/W at a keep-vein-open (KVO) rate
D. Should be started with D5/W at a maximum drip rate

4. For acute pulmonary edema of cardiac origin, morphine sulfate
    A. Is a drug of choice because it decreases venous return by acting as a pharmacological phlebotomizer, and also decreases anxiety levels
    B. Is classically contraindicated because it produces severe hypotension
    C. Is a drug of choice because it has significant inotropic effects on the myocardium and helps improve left ventricular function
    D. Decreases pulmonary alveolar-capillary permeability, thereby decreasing existing edema
    E. Decreases anxiety, decreases venous return, and may be given intravenously; also, its effects may be reversed by disopyramide phosphate (Norpace) if hypotension develops

5. Pitting pedal edema
    A. Is pathognomonic of heart failure
    B. Is directly correlated with the degree of pulmonary edema
    C. Can also be associated with renal or liver disease
    D. Is in itself a dangerous complication requiring immediate treatment

6. A significant laterally displaced apical pulse (PMI) indicates
    A. Severe emphysema
    B. Myocardial ischemia
    C. Cardiomegaly
    D. Constrictive pericarditis
    E. A congenital transposition of the great vessels
    F. None of the above

7. For your patient, a dopamine drip
    A. Is not advisable at this stage
    B. May lead to serious arrhythmias
    C. May be useful at a later point should signs of marked hypotension and hypoperfusion develop (assuming no arrhythmias are present)
    D. All of the above

8. Basic life support treatment of this patient may include
    A. Administration of high concentration oxygen
    B. Placement of the patient in the Trendelenburg position
    C. Use of ammonia inhalants to stimulate respiration
    D. Application of venous constricting bands
    E. Use of cool compresses to dilate peripheral vessels
    F. A and B are correct
    G. D and A are correct
    H. A, C, and D are correct

9. Your use of a lidocaine bolus accompanied by a lidocaine drip for treating the arrhythmia seen in your patient's initial EKG (Figure 9-1) must be carried out cautiously because of
    A. The possibility of a hypertensive episode
    B. The presence of congestive failure and a history of cirrhosis
    C. The demonstrated heart block
    D. The reported allergy to penicillin
    E. All of the above
    F. None of the above

10. Insertion of a Swan-Ganz catheter in your patient (by a physician at the hospital) will "classically" demonstrate
    A. An elevated right atrial pressure and an elevated pulmonary capillary wedge pressure
    B. Decreased pressures on both sides of the heart
    C. A low capillary wedge pressure with a high central venous pressure
    D. A high capillary wedge pressure with a low central venous pressure

11. The use of furosemide in your patient
    A. Has a primary inotropic effect
    B. May cause severe hyperkalemia
    C. Is contraindicated because of liver failure
    D. Is effective in selectively decreasing afterload
    E. Will serve as a slow-acting diuretic whose primary action is on the proximal tubules of the kidney
    F. May be effected by administration of a 400 mg bolus
    G. None of the above
    H. All of the above

12. Which of your patient's signs and symptoms are associated with left-sided heart failure?
    A. PND, cough, JVD
    B. JVD, HJR, peripheral edema
    C. PND, cough, orthopnea
    D. Ascites, cough, hepatomegaly
    E. PND, ascites, orthopnea

13. Your base physician inquires about the presence of fever, chills, rigors, and a productive cough. He may be considering the possibility of
    A. Acute pulmonary edema secondary to an acute myocardial infarction
    B. Esophageal varices
    C. Pleural effusion
    D. Pneumonia
    E. Pneumothorax

14. On admission to the emergency room, your patient is found to have an arterial blood pH of 7.21. This is most likely secondary to

A. Respiratory acidosis resulting from carbon dioxide retention
B. Metabolic acidosis resulting from carbon dioxide retention
C. Respiratory acidosis resulting from hypoxia
D. Metabolic acidosis of hyperglycemic origin
E. Respiratory alkalosis resulting from rapid respiratory rate and carbon dioxide blowoff
F. Metabolic acidosis resulting from buildup of lactic acid
G. Metabolic acidosis resulting from buildup of fumaric acid

Discussion

Acute pulmonary edema is a clinical condition characterized by excessive and dangerous levels of fluid accumulation in the lungs (Figure 9-2). This condition may be of cardiac origin (coronary heart disease, cardiomyopathies, valvular heart disease) or noncardiac origin (heroin, high altitudes, adult respiratory distress syndrome).

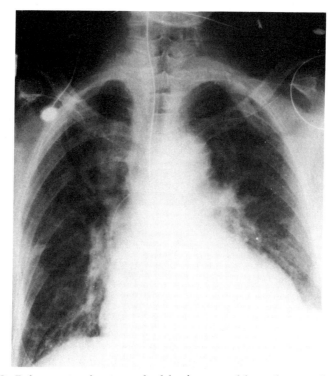

FIGURE 9-2. Pulmonary edema marked by increased bronchovascular markings, increased heart size, and left pleural effusion. (Cosgriff JH Jr, Anderson DL: The Practice of Emergency Care, 2nd ed, p 219. Philadelphia, JB Lippincott, 1984)

Acute pulmonary edema of cardiac origin occurs when the net forces causing transudation of fluid out of the capillaries and into the interstitial spaces and alveoli are greater than the forces removing fluid from the same area. This problem often occurs when disease processes result in impairment of left ventricular function. Increased pulmonary capillary permeability may also be a key factor in producing cardiac forms of pulmonary edema, though this mechanism of production is considered more characteristic of the noncardiac forms of pulmonary edema.

Since florid acute pulmonary edema is a late stage complication of heart failure, it is important to recognize the earlier signs and symptoms of myocardial dysfunction so that corrective measures may be taken. An important physical sign in your patient is the laterally displaced apical beat (PMI), which suggests cardiomegaly and serious cardiac pathology (Figure 9–3). Paroxysmal nocturnal dyspnea (awakening from sleep short of breath), orthopnea (dyspnea which is diminished when sitting up), and a cough (which may produce blood-tinged sputum), all present in your patient, are the result of pulmonary congestion and suggest underlying left-sided heart failure.

On the other hand, jugular venous distension (JVD), hepatojugular reflux (HJR), and ascites result from congestion in the systemic circulation and reflect right-sided heart failure. Although pitting edema does occur with heart failure, it is

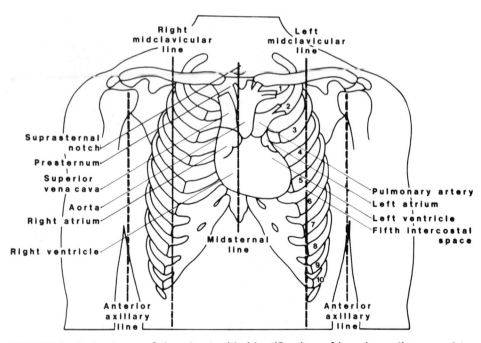

FIGURE 9–3. Anatomy of the chest with identification of imaginary lines used to describe findings. The normal location for the PMI is just medial to the left midclavicular line (MCL) at the 5th intercostal space (ICS). (Lamb JI, Carlson VR: Handbook of Cardiovascular Nursing, p 32. Philadelphia, JB Lippincott, 1986)

not necessarily diagnostic of that condition since it also occurs with liver disease, renal disease, and local vessel obstruction.

Before initiating treatment for pulmonary edema, other disease entities that may mimic this condition must be excluded. Pneumonia, for example, may present with abnormal breath sounds, cough, and dyspnea, all of which are also common to acute pulmonary edema. The two conditions can be differentiated by looking for fever, chills, productive cough, and pleuritic chest pain, all of which far more commonly accompany pneumonia. Given the absence of these signs, and the presence of serious cardiovascular symptomatology (JVD, HJR, PND), treatment should be based on a provisional field diagnosis of acute pulmonary edema secondary to *congestive heart failure* (CHF).

Treatment of your patient should include initial life support measures such as administering high concentration oxygen to correct hypoxia and to improve myocardial oxygenation; positioning the patient in an upright posture to ease breathing; and applying venous constricting bands to help decrease preload (this may be considered advanced life support in some localities). Advanced life support measures commence with establishing an intravenous line (IV) and include constant EKG monitoring. D5/W at a keep-vein-open (KVO) rate is the IV fluid of choice, because it may be administered without significantly increasing fluid load. EKG monitoring is important because patients with acute pulmonary edema often develop arrhythmias (premature ventricular contractions, sinus tachycardia, atrial fibrillation) due to marked hypoxemia, among other factors.

Initial drug therapy for pulmonary edema involves morphine sulfate and furosemide. Morphine sulfate acts to decrease ventricular afterload by lowering pressure and resistance in the arterial system and by decreasing preload (venous return). These combined actions help greatly in alleviating pulmonary congestion. Because morphine sulfate can cause respiratory depression and hypotension, it must be used cautiously and may not be advisable if pulmonary disease or hypotension preexist. In all cases where morphine is used, blood pressure should be measured repeatedly, and a drawn syringe of naloxone should be kept handy in case these adverse effects result.

Furosemide, a commonly used diuretic, works by impairing sodium chloride (and thus water) reabsorption from the ascending loop of Henle. Its usefulness in treating pulmonary edema is generally attributed to its ability to reduce blood volume and thereby help decrease preload. Its vasodilatory effects also help decrease venous return. It should be noted that this agent provides no significant direct inotropic or chronotropic actions on the heart. Although acute emergency use of furosemide in the field generally does not produce harmful side-effects, long-term use can result in hypokalemia unless the patient maintains adequate potassium intake.

Lidocaine is an important drug in controlling premature ventricular contractions (as seen in your patient), but must be used with great care in this case because of the patient's reported history of cirrhosis. The impaired liver function associated with cirrhosis may yield toxic serum levels of lidocaine due to the liver's inability to metabolize the drug. Signs of toxicity are primarily referable to the central nervous system and include seizures, psychotic behavior, and twitching.

Dopamine, a rapidly acting sympathomimetic drug, is used primarily to increase inotropicity and blood pressure. Since your patient is not in frank cardiogenic shock (*i.e.*, decreased blood pressure, increased pulse rate, and marked signs of organ hypoperfusion), the benefits of its use are far outweighed by the risks, which include cardiac arrhythmias and increased myocardial oxygen consumption.

More invasive diagnostic tests, including arterial blood gas measurement and hemodynamic monitoring, are necessary to better define your patient's status and will be carried out in the hospital. The pH of 7.21 indicates an acidosis, probably of metabolic origin and due to the buildup of lactic acid secondary to hypoxia.

Hemodynamic monitoring frequently involves using a Swan-Ganz catheter to measure right atrial pressure, right ventricular pressure, and pulmonary capillary wedge pressure. Your clinical findings of left-sided overload (*i.e.*, acute pulmonary edema) and the signs of right-sided overload (*i.e.*, JVD and HJR) are reflected in an elevated pulmonary capillary wedge pressure and right atrial pressure.

Field Diagnosis
- Cardiac arrhythmia
- Acute pulmonary edema
- Congestive heart failure

Hospital Diagnosis
- Congestive heart failure
- Acute myocardial infarction

Patient Follow-Up

The patient was admitted to the cardiac intensive care unit for careful monitoring and further evaluation. A full 12 lead EKG showed nonspecific ST elevations in the anterior leads, which is suggestive of an anterior wall myocardial infarct of undetermined age. Serial cardiac enzyme measurements also confirmed the diagnosis of an acute myocardial infarction. Your patient spent an uneventful 7 day course in the hospital and was then discharged.

Answers

1. A

    American Academy of Orthopaedic Surgeons: Emergency Care and Transportation of the Sick and Injured, 4th ed, p 316. Menasha, WI, George Banta Co, 1987

    Caroline NL: Emergency Care in the Streets, 3rd ed, pp 269–270. Boston, Little, Brown & Co, 1987

    Braunwald E: Heart failure. In Braunwald E, Isselbacher KJ, Petersdorf RG (eds): Harrison's Principles of Internal Medicine, 11th ed, p 907. New York, McGraw-Hill, 1987

2. D

    Huff J, Doernbach DP, White RD: ECG Workout: Exercises In Arrhythmia Interpretation, pp 138, 241 (strip 4.61). Philadelphia, JB Lippincott, 1985

3. **C**

Caroline NL: Emergency Care in the Streets, 3rd ed, p 269–270. Boston, Little, Brown & Co, 1987

American Heart Association: Standards and guidelines for cardiopulmonary resuscitation (CPR) and emergency cardiac care (ECC). JAMA 255:2905, (see page 2937), 1986

4. **A**

Caroline NL: Emergency Care in the Streets, 3rd ed, pp 148, 269–270. Boston, Little, Brown & Co, 1987

American Heart Association: Standards and guidelines for cardiopulmonary resuscitation (CPR) and emergency cardiac care (ECC). JAMA 255:2905, (see page 2938), 1986

5. **C**

Braunwald E: Edema. In Braunwald E, Isselbacher KJ, Petersdorf RG, (eds): Harrison's Principles of Internal Medicine, 11th ed, pp 149–153. New York, McGraw-Hill, 1987

6. **C**

O'Rourke RA, Braunwald E: Physical examination of the heart. In Braunwald E, Isselbacher KJ, Petersdorf RG (eds): Harrison's Principles of Internal Medicine, 11th ed, 867. New York, McGraw-Hill, 1987

7. **D**

Caroline NL: Emergency Care in the Streets, 3rd ed, pp 138–139, 269–272. Boston, Little, Brown & Co, 1987

American Heart Association: Standards and guidelines for cardiopulmonary resuscitation (CPR) and emergency cardiac care (ECC). JAMA 255:2905, (see page 2940–2941), 1986

8. **G**

American Academy of Orthopaedic Surgeons: Emergency Care and Transportation of the Sick and Injured, 4th ed, pp 315–317, 330. Menasha, WI, George Banta Co, 1987

American Heart Association: Standards and guidelines for cardiopulmonary resuscitation (CPR) and emergency cardiac care (ECC). JAMA 255:2905, (see page 2945), 1986

9. **B**

Caroline NL: Emergency Care in the Streets, 3rd ed, p 145. Boston, Little, Brown & Co, 1987

White RD: Lidocaine. EMT J 4:64, 1980

American Heart Association: Standards and guidelines for cardiopulmonary resuscitation (CPR) and emergency cardiac care (ECC). JAMA 255:2905, (see page 2938–2939), 1986

10. **A**

Caroline NL: Emergency Care in the Streets, 3rd ed, pp 269–271. Boston, Little, Brown & Co, 1987

Braunwald E: Normal and abnormal myocardial function. In Braunwald E, Isselbacher KJ, Petersdorf RG (eds): Harrison's Principles of Internal Medicine, 11th ed. New York, McGraw-Hill, 1987

Forrester JS, Diamond G, Chatterjee K, Swan HJC: Medical therapy of acute myocardial infarction by application of hemodynamic subsets. N Engl J Med 295:1356, 1976

11. **G**

Caroline NL: Emergency Care in the Streets, 3rd ed, pp 142–143, 270. Boston, Little, Brown & Co, 1987

Braunwald E: Heart failure. In Braunwald E, Isselbacher KJ, Petersdorf RG (eds): Harrison's Principles of Internal Medicine, 11th ed, 912–913. New York, McGraw-Hill, 1987

American Heart Association: Standards and guidelines for cardiopulmonary resuscitation (CPR) and emergency cardiac care (ECC). JAMA 255:2905, (see page 2942), 1986

12. **C**

American Academy of Orthopaedic Surgeons: Emergency Care and Transportation of the Sick and Injured, 4th ed, pp 316–317. Menasha, WI, George Banta Co, 1987

Caroline NL: Emergency Care in the Streets, 3rd ed, pp 269–271. Boston, Little, Brown & Co, 1987

Braunwald E: Heart failure. In Braunwald E, Isselbacher KJ, Petersdorf RG (eds): Harrison's Principles of Internal Medicine, 11th ed. New York, McGraw-Hill, 1987

13. **D**

Caroline NL: Emergency Care in the Streets, 3rd ed, p 208. Boston, Little, Brown & Co, 1987

14. **F**

Caroline NL: Emergency Care in the Streets, 3rd ed. p 71. Boston, Little, Brown & Co, 1987

Levinsky NG: Acidosis and Alkalosis. In Braunwald E, Isselbacher KJ, Petersdorf RG (eds): Harrison's Principles of Internal Medicine, 11th ed. New York, McGraw-Hill, 1987

Selected Reading

Clements SD Jr: Emergency evaluation and treatment of disorders resulting from coronary atherosclerotic heart disease. In Schwartz GR, Safar P, Stone JH, Storey PB, Wagner DK (eds): Principles and Practice of Emergency Medicine, 2nd ed, Philadelphia, WB Saunders, 1986
Codini MA: Management of acute myocardial infarction. Med Clin North Am 70:769, 1986
Robin ED, Cross CE, Zelis R: Pulmonary edema 2. N Engl J Med 288:292, 1973
Stapczynski JS: Myocardial ischemia and infarction: Heart failure. In Tintinalli JE, Rothstein RJ, Krome RL (eds): Emergency Medicine: A Comprehensive Study Guide. New York, McGraw-Hill, 1985
Ruggie N: Congestive heart failure. Med Clin North Am 70:829, 1986
Staub NC: The pathogenesis of pulmonary edema. Prog Cardiovasc Dis 23:53, 1980

TRAUMA EMERGENCIES

10

Acute Respiratory Distress Following a Stab Wound to the Chest

Your ambulance responds to a report of a "male stabbed." After a quick 5-minute response interval you pull up in front of a local bar. You are quickly led inside by police who direct you to a young man slumped in a chair clutching the right side of his chest. The patient relates that he became involved in a dispute and was stabbed once in the right side of his chest with a knife. He is fully conscious and complains of pain over the area of the stabbing and increasing shortness of breath.

As you begin your physical examination, you note that the patient is a 24-year-old man weighing approximately 160 pounds. He is conscious, and, although agitated, is able to answer your questions appropriately. He appears diaphoretic and in moderate respiratory distress. Vital signs are BP 100/72, pulse 120 and weak, respiration 24 shallow and labored, with a "hissing" noise heard over the chest during respiration. An EKG is recorded shortly after your arrival (Figure 10–1).

Head and neck examination are unremarkable; there is no evidence of trauma to the face or head and the trachea appears midline. The neck veins are not distended. Examination of the thorax reveals a moderate-size stab wound, measuring approximately 2 to 3 cm in length, in the third right intercostal space just medial to the midclavicular line. No evidence of rib fracture or subcutaneous emphysema is present. Respiratory excursion is markedly diminished on the affected side and auscultation reveals diminished-to-absent breath sounds over the right hemithorax. Percussion reveals dullness half the way up the right side, and a uniformly resonant note on the left side. Auscultation of the heart reveals clear sounds at a rate of 120 per minute. The abdomen is soft and nontender without evidence of trauma; bowel sounds are present. The extremities are cool, diaphoretic, and somewhat pallid; distal pulses are present and no gross trauma is evident. On neurologic examination the patient is alert and oriented to time, place, and person. He answers questions appropriately and shows no focal deficits. Motor and sensory function are grossly adequate in all extremities. There is no evidence of spinal cord injury.

You initiate treatment, contact medical control and measure vital signs again: BP 88/60, pulse 130 weak and irregular, and respiration 26 shallow and labored. Transport to a nearby medical facility begins.

106   *Trauma Emergencies*

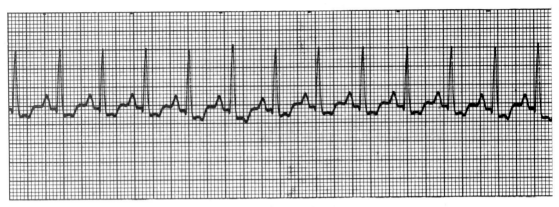

FIGURE 10-1. Lead II EKG recorded upon arrival at the scene.

Questions

Read each question carefully, keeping in mind the context of the case under discussion. Select the best answer from the choices presented.

1. Which of the following statements about a *flail chest* are correct?
    1. This condition involves fracture of several ribs (or the sternum) in more than one place
    2. The affected part of the chest wall often demonstrates "paradoxical motion" during breathing
    3. It is often (though not always) associated with a pneumothorax
    4. It is most commonly associated with dissection of the thoracic aorta

    A. 1, 2, and 3 are correct
    B. 1 and 3 are correct
    C. 2 and 4 are correct
    D. Only 4 is correct
    E. All are correct

2. Which of the following statements about *tension pneumothorax* are correct?
    1. It results from a one-way air leak into the pleural space which causes pressure to increase
    2. It may be accompanied by subcutaneous emphysema
    3. It frequently results in impaired venous return and decreased cardiac output
    4. It is characteristically associated with a shift of the mediastinum toward the injured side

    A. 1, 2, and 3 are correct
    B. 1 and 3 are correct
    C. 2 and 4 are correct
    D. Only 4 is correct
    E. All the above are correct

3. The term *pneumothorax* refers to
   A. Air within the lung
   B. Air within the pleural space
   C. Air within the chest wall and soft tissues
   D. Air within the pulmonary vasculature

4. Your patient's initial EKG (Figure 10-1) is best classified as
   A. Sinus tachycardia
   B. Junctional tachycardia
   C. Ventricular tachycardia
   D. Third degree AV block

5. Your patient is most likely suffering from
   1. Pneumothorax
   2. Tension pneumothorax
   3. Hemothorax
   4. Flail chest

   A. 1, 2, and 3 are correct
   B. 1 and 3 are correct
   C. 2 and 4 are correct
   D. Only 4 is correct
   E. All the above are correct

6. Your patient's treatment should include
   1. Constant cardiac monitoring
   2. Administering oxygen
   3. Establishing a large-bore intravenous line
   4. Covering the wound with petrolatum gauze

   A. 1, 2, and 3 are correct
   B. 1 and 3 are correct
   C. 2 and 4 are correct
   D. Only 4 is correct
   E. All the above are correct

Discussion

Chest injuries account for a major percentage of the deaths that result from trauma. Like abdominal trauma, chest trauma can be classified as *blunt* or *penetrating* depending on the mechanism and type of injury that results. The former is most frequently associated with motor vehicle accidents, the latter with stabbing and gunshot wounds.

In the present case, the young man's injury is obviously a penetrating injury to the right thorax at the level of the third interspace in the midclavicular line. Although it is not always feasible to do so, always attempt to gather the following basic facts in cases of penetrating chest trauma:

- Type of knife
- Length of blade
- Time elapsed since attack
- Whether the knife was impaled at any time
- How many times the patient recalls being stabbed
- Sex and size of attacker
- Angle at which the knife penetrated

Evaluate rapidly and conduct the standard primary survey to detect any life-threatening conditions. This patient has moderate respiratory distress, diminished breath sounds over the right hemithorax, dullness to percussion over the affected side, and a combination of tachycardia and hypotension. Analyzing these findings leads to a fairly good presumptive diagnosis. The findings of tachycardia and hypotension strongly suggest intravascular volume depletion. Because there is no evidence of external bleeding, it is likely that the patient is losing a significant amount of blood into his chest. The finding of dullness to percussion over the right hemithorax supports this belief. Based on this analysis you can conclude that the patient probably has a right *hemothorax*.

The patient's respiratory distress, lack of breath sounds in the right lung fields, and large penetrating chest wound suggest that the patient also has a right pneumothorax. The term *pneumothorax* simply denotes air in the pleural space. Several

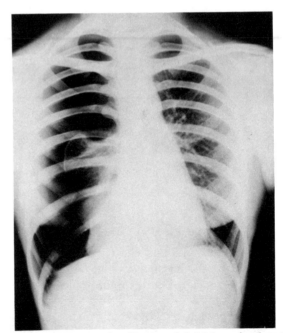

FIGURE 10-2. Pneumothorax. Total collapse of right lung is shown. Note that the mediastinal structures are shifted to the left. (Cosgriff JH Jr, Anderson DL: The Practice of Emergency Care, 2nd ed, p 357. Philadelphia, JB Lippincott, 1984)

Clinical Picture of Massive Pneumothorax and Hemothorax

PNEUMOTHORAX	HEMOTHORAX
Respiratory distress	Respiratory distress
Pleuritic chest pain	Pleuritic chest pain
Decreased breath sounds	Decreased breath sounds
Hyperresonance to percussion	Dullness to percussion
	Shock state
	• Hypotension
	• Tachycardia
	• Diaphoresis
Abnormal blood gases	Abnormal blood gases

types of pneumothoraces exist, but in all cases air accumulates in the pleural space, causing compression and collapse of the lung and preventing adequate respiration (Figure 10-2). In summary, your patient shows signs and symptoms that suggest he has sustained both a pneumothorax and a hemothorax (see "Clinical Picture of Massive Pneumothorax and Hemothorax").

As in most cases of major trauma, appropriate treatment involves supporting vital body functions and rapidly transporting the patient to a medical facility for definitive treatment. Rapidly seal your patient's chest wound, preferably with a sterile occlusive dressing, and administer supplemental oxygen. Establish at least one and, if feasible, two large-bore intravenous lines and administer a rapid infusion of normal saline or lactated Ringer's solution. Monitor vital signs and cardiac function while rapidly transporting the patient to a medical facility.

Field Diagnosis

- Pneumohemothorax
- Hypovolemic shock
- Cardiac arrhythmia

Hospital Diagnosis

- Pneumohemothorax
- Hemothorax
- Cardiac arrhythmia

Patient Follow-Up

Your patient was evaluated in the emergency room and found to have a large right pneumohemothorax. Aggressive management included placing a chest tube, after which the patient showed remarkable clinical improvement. After an uneventful hospital stay he was discharged, with advice from his physician to stay away from people with sharp pointed objects.

Answers

1. A
    Caroline NL: Emergency Care in the Streets, 3rd ed, pp 203–204. Boston, Little, Brown & Co, 1987
    Caroline NL: Emergency Medical Treatment: A Text for EMT-As and EMT-Intermediates, 2nd ed, pp 290–91. Boston, Little, Brown & Co, 1987

2. A
    Caroline NL: Emergency Care in the Streets, 3rd ed, pp 204–205. Boston, Little, Brown & Co, 1987
    Caroline NL: Emergency Medical Treatment: A Text for EMT-As and EMT-Intermediates, 2nd ed, pp 287–88. Boston, Little, Brown & Co, 1987
    American Academy of Orthopaedic Surgeons: Emergency Care and Transportation of the Sick and Injured, 4th ed, p 261. Menasha, WI, George Banta Co, 1987
    Grant HD, Murray RH Jr, Bergeron JD: Emergency Care, 4th ed, pp 310–313. Englewood Cliffs, NJ, Prentice-Hall, 1986

3. B
    Caroline NL: Emergency Care in the Streets, 3rd ed, p 204. Boston, Little, Brown & Co, 1987

4. A
    Huff J, Doernbach DP, White RD: ECG Workout: Exercises in Arrhythmia Interpretation, pp 27, 216 (strip 1.65). Philadelphia, JB Lippincott, 1985

5. B
    Caroline NL: Emergency Care in the Streets, 3rd ed, pp 200–207. Boston, Little, Brown & Co, 1987

6. E
    Caroline NL: Emergency Care in the Streets, 3rd ed, pp 200–207. Boston, Little, Brown & Co, 1987
    Caroline NL: Emergency Medical Treatment: A Text for EMT-As and EMT-Intermediates, 2nd ed, pp 287–295. Boston, Little, Brown & Co, 1987

Selected Reading

Cosgriff JH Jr, Anderson D: Thoracic and abdominal injuries. In Cosgriff JH Jr, Anderson DL: The Practice of Emergency Care, 2nd ed, Philadelphia, JB Lippincott, 1984

Jurkovich GJ, Moore EE: Hemothorax. In Edlich RF, Spyker DA, Haury BB (eds): Current Emergency Therapy, 3rd ed. Rockville, MD, Aspen Systems, 1986

Long WB: Penetrating chest trauma. In Edlich RF, Spyker DA, Haury BB (eds): Current Emergency Therapy, 3rd ed. Rockville, MD, Aspen Systems, 1986

Rubio PA: Pneumothorax. In Edlich RF, Spyker DA, Haury BB (eds): Current Emergency Therapy, 3rd ed. Rockville, MD, Aspen Systems, 1986

Wilson RF, Steiger Z: Thoracic injuries. In Tintinalli JE, Rothstein RJ, Krome RL (eds): Emergency Medicine: A Comprehensive Study Guide. New York, McGraw-Hill, 1985

11

Orthopedic Injuries in a Multiple Trauma Victim

You and your partner respond to a report of a "man struck by an auto." After a short response interval, you pull up along the shoulder of a major highway where you are greeted by police, fire, and emergency service workers. Traffic has been detoured and you are directed to the far right lane of a three lane highway where you find a young man lying face up on the ground. Rescue workers inform you that the gentleman attempted to cross the highway and was struck by an oncoming vehicle.

The patient is a 22-year-old man weighing approximately 180 pounds; he is conscious and breathing spontaneously. Vital signs are BP 116/76 (left arm, supine), pulse 120 and regular, and respiration 18 and regular. Head and neck examination reveals multiple abrasions over the face, a 2 cm laceration just above the right ear, and several small lacerations over the forehead. The trachea appears midline and there is no evidence of fracture over the skull. The ears, nose, and oropharynx are free of foreign debris, blood, and other fluid. The thorax is without deformity, respiratory excursion is symmetrical, and breath sounds are clear bilaterally. Heart sounds are S_1S_2 and clear at a regular rate of 120 beats per minute.

The abdomen has multiple abrasions and is rigid and painful to palpation; bowel sounds cannot be auscultated. Examination of the musculoskeletal system reveals significant pain and instability upon compression of the iliac crests, but no protruding bone fragments. On further examination, you note marked deformity, swelling, and pain over the distal one third of the right forearm, but no open wounds or protruding bone fragments. A distal pulse is palpated, the right hand has good color, and the hand is warm to touch.

Neurologic examination indicates that the patient is conscious but extremely agitated. He opens his eyes spontaneously and is oriented to time, place, and person. Pupils are round, equal, and reactive to light. Palpation shows the cervical and lower spine to be without gross deformity, although you note point tenderness and paravertebral muscle spasm over both the lower cervical and upper thoracic vertebrae. Priapism is not noted and the patient is continent of urine and feces. Spontaneous movement is present in all extremities but is seriously impaired in the distal right limb; sensation is present in all extremities, over the thorax, and over the abdomen. Vital signs repeated 5 minutes after arrival reveal the following: BP

100/70 (left arm, supine), pulse 140 weak and regular, and respiration 28 and regular.

You initiate treatment, contact medical control, and begin transport.

Questions

Read each question carefully, keeping in mind the context of the case at hand. Select the best answer from the choices presented.

1. Your patient's vital signs suggest
   A. Marked intravascular volume depletion
   B. Normal intravascular volume
   C. Increased intravascular volume
   D. None of the above

2. Your abdominal examination suggests
   A. Acute appendicitis
   B. Acute rupture of the aorta
   C. Intraabdominal hemorrhage
   D. Spontaneous bacterial peritonitis

3. Complications that may be seen with pelvic fractures include
   1. Blood loss into the retroperitoneal space
   2. Hypovolemic shock
   3. Injury to the urinary bladder
   4. Hematuria

   A. 1, 2, and 3 are correct
   B. 1 and 3 are correct
   C. 2 and 4 are correct
   D. Only 4 is correct
   E. All are correct

4. The pelvic bone is formed by the union of the
   1. Ilium
   2. Pubis
   3. Ischium
   4. Clinoid

   A. 1, 2, and 3 are correct
   B. 1 and 3 are correct
   C. 2 and 4 are correct
   D. Only 4 is correct
   E. All are correct

5. Important structures and relations of the pelvis include

A. Sacrum, two pelvic bones, symphysis pubis, sacroiliac joints
b. Three pelvic bones, symphysis pubis, sacropubic joint, sacrum
C. Two pelvic bones, sacroischial joints, symphysis pubis, sacrum
D. Six pelvic bones, acetabulum, sacropubic joint, xiphoid

6. Bony structures of the forearm include
   1. Radius
   2. Humerus
   3. Ulna
   4. Clavicle

   A. 1, 2, and 3 are correct
   B. 1 and 3 are correct
   C. 2 and 4 are correct
   D. Only 4 is correct
   E. All are correct

7. Correct management of your patient should be based on a field diagnosis of which of the following?
   1. Pelvic fracture
   2. Intraabdominal injury
   3. Forearm fracture
   4. Spinal injury

   A. 1, 2, and 3 are correct
   B. 1 and 3 are correct
   C. 2 and 4 are correct
   D. Only 4 is correct
   E. All are correct

8. Splinting devices that may be used to treat your patient include a
   1. "Long board" for immobilization
   2. Rigid splint applied to the upper right limb
   3. Cervical collar
   4. Traction splint

   A. 1, 2, and 3 are correct
   B. 1 and 3 are correct
   C. 2 and 4 are correct
   D. Only 4 is correct
   E. All are correct

9. Basic life support should include
   1. Administration of supplemental oxygen
   2. Complete spinal immobilization
   3. Frequent monitoring of vital signs
   4. Application of MAST

A. 1, 2, and 3 are correct
B. 1 and 3 are correct
C. 2 and 4 are correct
D. Only 4 is correct
E. All are correct

10. Advanced life support treatment might include
    1. Establishing an intravenous line
    2. Administering lactated Ringer's
    3. Cardiac monitoring
    4. Administering atropine

    A. 1, 2, and 3 are correct
    B. 1 and 3 are correct
    C. 2 and 4 are correct
    D. Only 4 is correct
    E. All are correct

Discussion

In the present scenario we are faced with a trauma patient with multiple injuries. Proper management of such a patient includes a rapid but complete evaluation, adequate supportive treatment, and rapid transport to a medical facility. Initial assessment starts, of course, with the standard "ABCs": A = airway, B = breathing, C = circulation and cervical spine. Only with these areas properly managed can further evaluation and treatment continue. In this patient the airway appears intact, breathing is adequate, and there is no evidence of external life-threatening hemorrhage. Rapid assessment of the cervical spine reveals marked point tenderness and muscle spasm, both of which, in the setting of major trauma, suggest the definite possibility of cervical spine injury. Gentle traction and immediate application of a cervical collar are indicated.

The next step in patient management is measuring vital signs and performing a rapid secondary survey. The patient's initial vital signs (BP 116/76, pulse 120 and regular, respiration 18 and regular) are notable for an unusually rapid pulse rate, a finding which begs explanation and should raise the suspicion of intravascular volume depletion secondary to hypovolemic shock. Although the blood pressure appears normal (116/76), we do not know the patient's baseline blood pressure. This value, if known, might portray the present reading in a different light; if, for instance, his normal blood pressure is 130/88, then the present reading of 116/76 would be abnormal. Also, hypotension is a relatively late indicator of hypovolemic shock; tachycardia and other signs appear long before (see "Clinical Manifestations of Hypovolemic Shock"). The best course of action is to presume that early hypovolemic shock is present and carry out serial measurements of both pulse and blood pressure.

The secondary survey reveals several significant findings, mostly concerning the gastrointestinal, musculoskeletal, and neurologic systems. Abdominal rigidity,

Clinical Manifestations of Hypovolemic Shock

- Pallor
- Diaphoresis
- Oliguria or anuria
- Tachycardia
- Restlessness
- Agitation
- Altered mental state
- Relative or absolute hypotension

pain, and decreased or absent bowel sounds strongly suggest major intraabdominal injury. Since there is no evidence of penetrating trauma, one must conclude that the patient has sustained significant blunt abdominal trauma resulting in major internal injury. These physical findings, considered in the context of a falling blood pressure and a rising pulse rate (signs of hypovolemic shock), strongly intimate that there may be ongoing intraabdominal bleeding. Although the source of injury cannot be known without further evaluation, among the most common organs to suffer injury in cases of blunt trauma are the spleen and liver. Proper treatment includes rapidly establishing at least one, and preferably two, large-bore intravenous (IV) lines, and then rapidly administering a suitable replacement fluid such as lactated Ringer's or normal saline. Also apply military antishock trousers (MAST) and inflate if local protocols and the patient's clinical status require.

The musculoskeletal assessment also reveals several major injuries that require treatment. The pelvis is made up of three bones: the two pelvic bones (each formed by the union of the ilium, ischium, and pubis) and the sacrum. The sacrum articulates on each side with one of the two pelvic bones via the sacroiliac joint and the two pelvic bones in turn join anteriorly in the midline at the symphysis pubis. Together these bones form a sturdy ringlike structure. The physical findings in your patient of severe pain and instability upon compression of the iliac crests strongly suggest a pelvic fracture. Because such a fracture may result in significant blood loss as well as damage to adjacent structures (*e.g.,* rupture of the bladder), it must be carefully managed. Immobilize the patient with a "longboard" and if he shows signs of hypovolemia (as in the present case) apply MAST. Military antishock trousers serve several important functions: they stabilize the fracture, tampon bleeding, and elevate blood pressure.

This patient also suffers serious deformity, swelling, and pain in the distal right forearm. Since the principal bony structures that make up the forearm include the radius and the ulna, either or both of these bones may be fractured. It is important in such injuries to evaluate the distal extremity and ensure that there is adequate neurovascular function. Check for sensation, presence of a distal pulse, and color and temperature of the distal extremity. Splinting should be carried out according to the general rule stipulating "one joint above and one joint below" the site of injury. Use a rigid board splint or air splint.

Neurologic evaluation of this patient reveals cervical and thoracic spine point tenderness. These conditions are best handled by complete spinal immobilization. As with any major trauma case, frequent reassessment of the patient's neurologic status is mandatory.

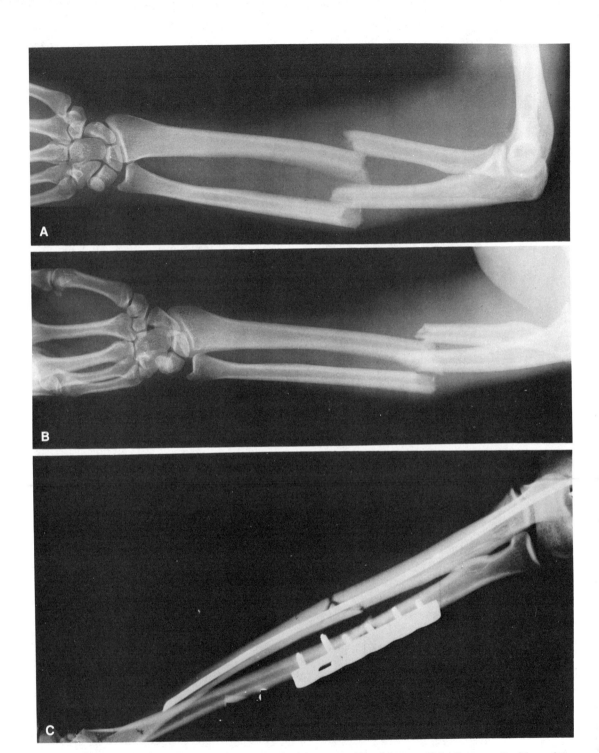

FIGURE 11-1. (*A* and *B*) Displaced fractures of both bones of the forearm. Position of the fragments is the result of muscle tension in the forearm, causing displacement and overriding of the bone ends (shortening). (*C*) Treatment by open reduction and internal fixation, seen by postoperative x-ray, resulted in good position of the fragments. (Cosgriff JH Jr, Anderson DL: The Practice of Emergency Care, 2nd ed, p 582. Philadelphia, JB Lippincott, 1984)

> **Field Diagnosis**
> - Multiple organ system trauma
>
> **Hospital Diagnosis**
> - Pelvic fracture
> - Fracture of radius and ulna
> - Splenic rupture
> - Hypovolemic shock

Patient Follow-Up

After arriving at the emergency room your patient continued to demonstrate signs of progressive intravascular volume loss and increasing abdominal rigidity. An exploratory laparotomy was performed and confirmed the suspicion of splenic rupture. A splenectomy was performed. Additional evaluation revealed a displaced fracture of the forearm, which was managed by open reduction and internal fixation (Figure 11-1), as well as an unstable pelvic fracture.

Answers

1. A
   Grant HD, Murray RH Jr, Bergeron JD: Emergency Care, 4th ed, pp 167-174. Englewood Cliffs, NJ, Prentice-Hall, 1986
   American Academy of Orthopaedic Surgeons: Emergency Care and Transportation of the Sick and Injured, 4th ed, p 138. Menasha, WI, George Banta Co, 1987
   Caroline NL: Emergency Care in the Streets, 3rd ed, pp 78-82. Boston, Little, Brown & Co, 1987

2. C
   American Academy of Orthopaedic Surgeons: Emergency Care and Transportation of the Sick and Injured, 4th ed, pp 276-279. Menasha, WI, George Banta Co, 1987
   Caroline NL: Emergency Care in the Streets, 3rd ed, pp 397-399. Boston, Little, Brown & Co, 1987

3. E
   American Academy of Orthopaedic Surgeons: Emergency Care and Transportation of the Sick and Injured, 4th ed, pp 205-207. Menasha, WI, George Banta Co, 1987
   Grant HD, Murray RH Jr, Bergeron JD: Emergency Care, 4th ed, p 233. Englewood Cliffs, NJ, Prentice-Hall, 1986.
   Caroline NL: Emergency Medical Treatment: A Text for EMT-As and EMT-Intermediates, 2nd ed, pp 330-332. Boston, Little, Brown & Co, 1987

4. A
   American Academy of Orthopaedic Surgeons: Emergency Care and Transportation of the Sick and Injured, 4th ed, p 29. Menasha, WI, George Banta Co, 1987
   Caroline NL: Emergency Medical Treatment: A Text for EMT-As and EMT-Intermediates, 2nd ed, p 313. Boston, Little, Brown & Co, 1987
   Caroline NL: Emergency Care in the Streets, 3rd ed, p 25. Boston, Little, Brown & Co, 1987

5. A
   American Academy of Orthopaedic Surgeons: Emergency Care and Transportation of the Sick and Injured, 4th ed, p 29. Menasha, WI, George Banta Co, 1987
   Caroline NL: Emergency Medical Treatment: A Text for EMT-As and EMT-In-

termediates, 2nd ed, p 313. Boston, Little, Brown & Co, 1987

Caroline NL: Emergency Care in the Streets, 3rd ed, p 25. Boston, Little, Brown & Co, 1987

6. B

Caroline NL: Emergency Medical Treatment: A Text for EMT-As and EMT-Intermediates, 2nd ed, p 24. Boston, Little, Brown & Co, 1987

Caroline NL: Emergency Care in the Streets, 3rd ed, p 23. Boston, Little, Brown & Co, 1987

7. E

Caroline NL: Emergency Care in the Streets, 3rd ed, pp 51, 397-399, 409-410. Boston, Little, Brown & Co, 1987

8. E

American Academy of Orthopaedic Surgeons: Emergency Care and Transportation of the Sick and Injured, 4th ed, pp 202-203. Menasha, WI, George Banta Co, 1987

Caroline NL: Emergency Care in the Streets. 3rd ed, pp 370-371, 413-418. Boston, Little, Brown & Co, 1987

9. E

American Academy of Orthopaedic Surgeons: Emergency Care and Transportation of the Sick and Injured, 4th ed, pp 187-194, 205-207. Menasha, WI, George Banta Co, 1987

Caroline NL: Emergency Medical Treatment: A Text for EMT-As and EMT-Intermediates, 2nd ed, p 306. Boston, Little, Brown & Co, 1987

10. A

Caroline NL: Emergency Care in the Streets, 3rd ed, pp 80-81. Boston, Little, Brown & Co, 1987

Selected Reading

Blaisdell FW, Trunkey DD (eds): Trauma Management: Abdominal Trauma. New York, Thieme-Stratton, 1982

Fitch RD: Fractures and dislocations of the shoulder, arm, and forearm. In Sabiston DC Jr (ed): Textbook of Surgery, 13th ed. Philadelphia, WB Saunders, 1986

Harrelson JM: Fractures and dislocations: general principles. In Sabiston DC Jr (ed): Textbook of Surgery, 13th ed. Philadelphia, WB Saunders, 1986

McCollum DE: Fractures of the pelvis, femur, and knee. In Sabiston DC Jr (ed): Textbook of Surgery, 13th ed. Philadelphia, WB Saunders, 1986

Shires TG, Canizaro PC, Carrico CJ: Shock. In Schwartz SI (ed): Principles of Surgery, 4th ed. New York, McGraw-Hill, 1984

12

Penetrating Abdominal Trauma in a Young Man

Your ambulance responds to a report of a "male shot." After a rapid response you arrive at the scene where you notice a large crowd has gathered. After securing the vehicle and gathering your equipment, you are guided through the crowd by a police officer who tells you that the victim was "shot in the stomach." You approach the man, who is lying face up in a small pool of blood; while the police contain the crowd, you and your partner begin evaluating the patient.

The patient is a young man in his middle 20s who weighs approximately 160 pounds. He is conscious and breathing spontaneously. Initial inspection reveals a small-caliber gunshot wound to the abdomen. An initial set of vital signs, measured with the patient in a supine position, indicates the following: BP 88 by palpation, pulse 110 regular and weak, and respiration 24 shallow and regular. Cardiac monitoring at this time reveals the tracing shown below (Figure 12-1).

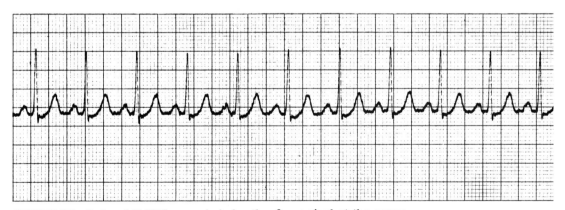

FIGURE 12-1. Lead II EKG recorded shortly after arrival at the scene.

On physical examination the head and neck show no signs of trauma and the trachea is midline. The conjunctiva are pallid and the pupils appear round, equal, and reactive to light. No blood or cerebrospinal fluid are seen draining from the nose or external auditory canals. The thorax is symmetrical and respiratory excursion is somewhat diminished. Palpation reveals no indications of fractures or deformity. Auscultation of the anterior lung fields indicates bilateral breath sounds without rhonchi, rales, or wheezes. Heart sounds are S_1S_2; they are clear but somewhat diminished in intensity. On inspection the abdomen shows a single, small-caliber gunshot entrance wound located 1 to 2 inches below the xiphoid process. No active external bleeding is noted. No exit wound can be found. The abdomen is "rock hard" to palpation and bowel sounds are not heard.

Examination of the extremities and pelvic girdle reveals no evidence of fractures or deformity. On neurologic examination your patient is conscious although combative; he is uncooperative, appears somewhat disoriented, and is unable to respond clearly to questions asked of him. You note spontaneous movements in the upper extremities but none in the lower extremities. A quick attempt to evaluate for sensation and motor strength is unsuccessful because the patient will not cooperate.

Medical control is contacted while appropriate field treatment is carried out. Vital signs repeated during transport to the hospital and after initiation of treatment are BP 90/60, pulse 130 regular and weak, and respiration 28 shallow and regular. Cardiac monitoring at this point reveals the following (Figure 12-2).

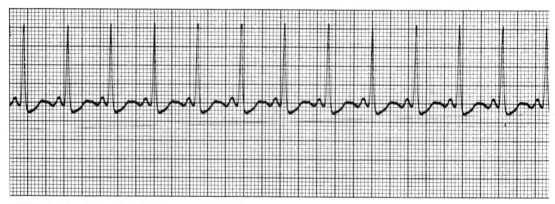

FIGURE 12-2. Lead II EKG recorded during transport to the hospital.

When you arrive at the hospital, the physician in charge orders the following tests and measurements: arterial blood gas, complete blood count, serum electrolytes, serum glucose, blood urea nitrogen (BUN), urinalysis, coagulation studies, and type and crossmatch. Chest and abdominal radiographs are also obtained.

Questions

Read each question carefully, keeping in mind the context of the case under discussion. Select the best answer from the choices presented.

1. For purposes of localization, the external surface of the abdomen may be divided into nine regions. These include all of the following except
   A. Right hypochondriac

B. Left lumbar
   C. Umbilical
   D. Left digastric

2. The point of entrance of the bullet is best described as being in the
   A. Hypogastric region at the level of the body of the fifth lumbar vertebra (L5)
   B. Epigastric region at the level of the body of the twelfth thoracic vertebra (T12)
   C. Infrasternal angle at the level of the body of the sixth thoracic vertebra (T6)
   D. Hypogastric region at the level of the body of the second lumbar vertebra (L2)

3. Treatment of your patient is best based upon a field diagnosis of
   A. Cardiogenic shock
   B. Septic shock
   C. Neurogenic shock
   D. Anaphylactic shock
   E. Hypovolemic shock

4. Although not frequently seen, a physical finding associated with massive hemorrhage into the abdominopelvic cavity is
   A. Yellow green discoloration over the xiphoid region
   B. Purple red discoloration over the left iliac fossa
   C. Blue grey discoloration over the umbilical region
   D. Red orange discoloration over the xiphoid region

5. Which of the following has the greatest muzzle velocity?
   A. .22 Magnum
   B. .38 Colt
   C. .270 Winchester
   D. .357 Magnum

6. Basic life support treatment of your patient should include which of the following?
   1. Administration of high-concentration oxygen
   2. Rapid spinal immobilization on a "long backboard"
   3. Application of a sterile bandage and dressing
   4. Alcohol irrigation of the abdominal wound

   A. 1, 2, and 3 are correct
   B. 1 and 3 are correct
   C. 2 and 4 are correct
   D. Only 4 is correct
   E. All are correct

7. Advanced life support treatment of this patient should include which of the following procedures?

1. Establishment of a large-bore intravenous line
2. Endotracheal intubation
3. Application of MAST
4. Administration of D5/W at a "wide open" rate

A. 1, 2, and 3 are correct
B. 1 and 3 are correct
C. 2 and 4 are correct
D. Only 4 is correct
E. All are correct

8. The results of the type and crossmatch test indicate that your patient's blood type is A and that he is Rh positive. Which of the following blood types is suitable for transfusion?
   1. A positive
   2. B positive
   3. O negative
   4. AB positive

   A. 1, 2, and 3 are correct
   B. 1 and 3 are correct
   C. 2 and 4 are correct
   D. Only 4 is correct
   E. All are correct

9. When compared with your patient's initial vital signs, those taken during transport (after the initiation of treatment) suggest that
   A. Internal bleeding has, for the most part, stopped
   B. Substantial internal bleeding is still occurring
   C. The information given provides no clues about the extent of blood loss

Discussion

This patient is suffering from hypovolemic shock secondary to a penetrating abdominal trauma resulting from a small-caliber gunshot wound.

The external abdominopelvic wall may be divided into nine regions for purposes of localization. These regions are mapped out by plotting the subcostal and transtubercular planes horizontally and the right and left midclavicular lines vertically. The resulting points of intersection delineate nine regions:

- Epigastric
- Right and left hypochondriac
- Umbilical
- Right and left lumbar
- Hypogastric
- Right and left iliac

Because the spatial relationships of the abdominal viscera, both to each other and to the body surface, are generally described with respect to the vertebral column, it is important to understand the correspondence between various points on the external abdominal wall and their respective vertebral levels. The various vertebral levels may be defined by a series of horizontal planes running across the abdomen (Table 12–1).

Knowledge of the nine abdominal regions and the vertebral levels allows the paramedic to describe the bullet's point of entrance in a clear and exact fashion. In the case at hand, the bullet entered the abdomen 1 to 2 inches below the xiphoid. Its point of penetration is thus in the epigastric region, just above the transpyloric plane (L1/L2 vertebral level) and hence, at approximately the twelfth thoracic vertebra.

Before describing the compensatory cardiovascular mechanisms brought into play by your patient's injuries, a review of some key terms is in order:

- *Cardiac output* = stroke volume × heart rate
- *Stroke volume* = the volume of blood pumped by the ventricle with each contraction
- *Venous return* = the volume of blood flowing into the right atrium each minute
- *Mean systemic filling pressure* = the effective pressure which tends to force blood back to the heart; it reflects the degree of filling of the vascular system

In the present case, the patient's hypotensive state and increasing tachycardia indicate internal hemorrhage. Loss of blood from the vascular system reduces the degree of filling; hence, mean systemic filling pressure falls. Because this is the major driving force pushing blood back to the right atrium, there is also a decrease in venous return. Since the amount of blood pumped out of the heart with each contraction (stroke volume) is obviously limited by the amount of blood returning to the heart (venous return), decreased stroke volume also results. In summary,

TABLE 12–1. Topographical Anatomy of the Abdomen

Plane	Location	Corresponding Vertebral Level
Transpyloric	Runs horizontally across abdomen at a point midway between xiphisternal joint and the umbilicus	At the intervertebral disc between L1 and L2 vertebrae
Subcostal	Runs horizontally across abdomen, joining the lowest points of the costal margin on each side	At the intervertebral disc between L2 and L3
Transumbilical	Runs horizontally across abdomen, passing through umbilicus	At the intervertebral disc between L3 and L4
Transtubercular	Runs horizontally across abdomen and passes through the iliac tubercules	At the body of L5 vertebra
Supracristal	Runs horizontally, passing across the top of iliac crests	At the level of L4 vertebra

(Greenberg MD, Lieber JJ: Penetrating trauma. J Emerg Care Trans Sept/Oct: 74, 1984)

your patient's clinical condition is characterized physiologically by a decreased stroke volume and decreased mean systemic filling pressure.

The resulting low-output, hypovolemic state calls into play several compensatory mechanisms that attempt to maintain an adequate cardiac output, blood pressure, and tissue perfusion. The falling blood pressure is sensed by baroreceptors located in the carotid sinuses and aortic arch. They stimulate the vasoconstrictor center in the medulla, which in turn causes sympathetic vasoconstriction and an increase in heart rate and strength of contraction. Additionally, the tendency of the vessels (especially the veins) to decrease their overall volume-holding capacity and "tighten up" around the remaining vascular contents helps raise the intravascular pressure. This process is known as *reverse stress relaxation.*

Other compensatory mechanisms involve the release of various hormones. Epinephrine and norepinephrine are released by the adrenal medulla into the blood and further enhance vasoconstriction and cardiac performance. Renin is secreted by the juxtaglomerular cells of the kidney and acts upon a plasma protein to form angiotensin I. This, in turn, is converted (primarily in the lungs) to angiotensin II, whose immediate action is to help elevate total peripheral resistance by causing vasoconstriction.

Treatment of this patient should be aimed at correcting his deteriorating hemodynamic status. Additionally, the lack of spontaneous movements in the lower extremities suggests the possibility of traumatic spinal cord injury. Basic life support measures include bandaging, oxygen administration, placement on a "long backboard," and conservation of body heat. Irrigating the abdominal wound with alcohol is dangerous and unnecessary. Placing the patient in a sitting position is inadvisable because of the existing hypotension and the distinct possibility of spinal cord injury. Advanced life support treatment should include applying military antishock trousers (MAST), establishing a large-bore intravenous line, and administering Ringer's lactate, normal saline, or another suitable volume replacement solution.

Field Diagnosis

- Penetrating abdominal trauma
- Hypovolemic shock
- Spinal cord injury
- Cardiac arrhythmia

Hospital Diagnosis

- Penetrating abdominal injury
- Hypovolemic shock
- Spinal cord injury

Patient Follow-Up

The patient was quickly evaluated in the emergency room and then taken to the operating room. Surgical exploration revealed significant injury to the stomach, pancreas, liver, and small intestine, but no penetration of the diaphragm. The bullet was found lodged against the spinal column in the upper lumbar region. Following a prolonged postoperative recovery, the patient recovered and regained full motor and sensory function in his lower extremities.

Answers

1. D

    Moore KL: Clinically Oriented Anatomy, 2nd ed, p 155. Baltimore, Williams & Wilkins, 1985

2. B

    Moore KL: Clinically Oriented Anatomy, 2nd ed, pp 61, 155. Baltimore, Williams & Wilkins, 1985

3. E

    Caroline NL: Emergency Care in the Streets, 3rd ed, pp 78–83. Boston, Little, Brown & Co, 1987

    Caroline NL: Emergency Medical Treatment: A Text for EMT-As and EMT-Intermediates, 2nd ed, pp 405–406. Boston, Little, Brown & Co, 1987

4. C

    Caroline NL: Emergency Care in the Streets, 3rd ed, p 398. Boston, Little, Brown & Co, 1987

5. C

    Blaisdell FW, Trunkey DD (eds): Trauma Management: Abdominal Trauma, p 3. New York, Thieme-Stratton, 1982

    Wilson JM: Shotgun ballistics and shotgun injuries. West J Med 129:149–155, 1978

6. A

    Caroline NL: Emergency Care in the Streets, 3rd ed, pp 80–83, 89–91, 397–402. Boston, Little, Brown & Co, 1987

    Caroline NL: Emergency Medical Treatment: A Text for EMT-As and EMT-Intermediates, 2nd ed, pp 305–306. Boston, Little, Brown & Co, 1987

    Grant HD, Murray RH Jr, Bergeron JD: Emergency Care, 4th ed, p 320. Englewood Cliffs, NJ, Prentice-Hall, 1986

7. A

    Caroline NL: Emergency Care in the Streets, 3rd ed, pp 80–83, 89–91, 397–402. Boston, Little, Brown & Co, 1987

    Caroline NL: Emergency Medical Treatment: A Text for EMT-As and EMT-Intermediates, 2nd ed, pp 305–06. Boston, Little, Brown & Co, 1987

8. B

    Caroline NL: Emergency Care in the Streets, 3rd ed, pp 73–74. Boston, Little, Brown & Co, 1987

    Collins JA: Blood transfusions and disorders of surgical bleeding. In Sabiston DC Jr (ed): Textbook of Surgery, 13th ed. Philadelphia, WB Saunders, 1986

9. B

    See discussion for explanation.

Selected Reading

Blaisdell FW, Trunkey DD (eds): Trauma Management: Abdominal Trauma, p 3. New York, Thieme-Stratton, 1982

Conn AT: Hypovolemic shock. Emerg Care Quarterly 1:37, 1985

Holcroft JW, Blaisdell FW: Shock: Causes and management of circulatory collapse. In Sabiston DC Jr (ed): Textbook of Surgery, 13th ed. Philadelphia, WB Saunders, 1986

Jacobs BB, Jacobs LM: Prehospital resuscitation of the trauma patient. Top Emerg Med 9:1, 1987

Oreskovich MR, Carrico CJ: Trauma: Management of the acutely injured patient. In Sabiston DC Jr (ed): Textbook of Surgery, 13th ed. Philadelphia, WB Saunders, 1986

13

Thermal Injuries in a 28-Year-Old Man

Your ambulance is dispatched to the scene of an industrial fire. As you pull up, the police direct you to the exact location and you secure your vehicle a safe distance away. After making your way through the crowd, you are directed to a vacant park across the street from the scene of the fire, where you see a badly burned man in his late twenties lying on the ground, apparently conscious and in severe pain. A firefighter is holding an oxygen mask over the patient's face. As you start your primary survey, the firefighter tells you that your patient was found unconscious in a small back room with his shirt on fire. Further questioning reveals that the building contained assorted drums of unknown chemicals and that, upon arrival, the firefighter encountered a heavy smoke condition. You begin working on your patient, while your partner gathers more information from bystanders.

Your patient is a 28-year-old man weighing 175 pounds. He complains of severe pain and shortness of breath and, although conscious, appears somewhat confused. His initial set of vital signs are BP 180/100 supine (orthostatics not taken due to patient condition), pulse 80 and irregular, respiration 40 regular and shallow, and body temperature cool to touch.

Your physical examination indicates no signs of gross trauma to the patient's head. His pupils are round, equal, and reactive to light. The mouth and throat show generalized erythema and swelling. The face shows singeing of the eyebrows, eyelashes, and hair. The entire face is covered with erythematous, blistering burns sensitive to touch. The cervical spine shows no apparent deformity or point tenderness. A thoracic examination reveals painful, erythematous, blistering burns over the entire anterior trunk.

Respiratory excursion appears symmetrical. Observation of the thorax indicates no gross deformity or abnormalities. Palpation is deferred due to the patient's extreme pain. Auscultation (in supine position) reveals diffuse bilateral inspiratory and expiratory wheezes with rhonchi. Diminished breath sounds at the base of both lungs are noted.

Heart sounds are clear and crisp with normal S1S2. The genitalia show no evidence of injury or burns. Injuries to the extremities include charring over both the right and left palmar surfaces and over the left anterior forearm. The remaining skin appears unremarkable. No edema is noted. Distal pulses are present and equal.

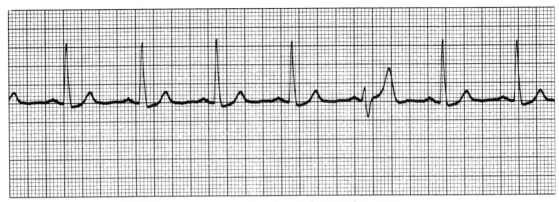

FIGURE 13-1. Lead II EKG recorded shortly after arrival at the scene.

No gross fractures or deformities are observable. A cursory neurologic examination reveals no gross focal findings.

The patient is placed on an EKG monitor and a lead II 6-second strip is recorded (Figure 13-1). You begin appropriate field treatment, contact medical control, and report an estimated time of arrival at the hospital of 45 minutes. In transit, your patient remains stable and a second EKG strip is recorded (Figure 13-2). Vital signs are monitored at 5-minute intervals.

Upon your arrival in the emergency room, the following tests are performed immediately: arterial blood gas (ABG), complete blood count (CBC) with differential and platelet count, serum electrolytes, serum glucose, blood urea nitrogen (BUN), creatinine, urinalysis, coagulation studies, type and crossmatch, arterial carboxyhemoglobin, and serum and urine myoglobin. In addition, emergency chest and abdominal radiographs are obtained (see "Laboratory Results").

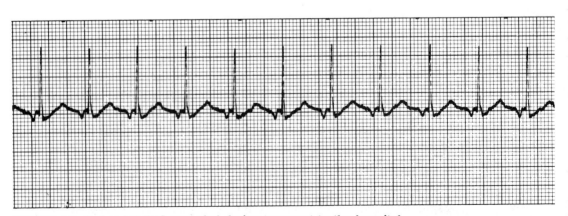

FIGURE 13-2. Lead II EKG recorded during transport to the hospital.

Laboratory Results

Chemistries

- ABG: pH 7.52, Po_2 210 mmHg, PCo_2 22 mmHg
- CBC: WBC 18.2×10^3 cu mm, Hb 17 g/dl, Hct 48%, platelets normal
- Serum electrolytes: K^+ 5.3 mEq/L, Na^+ 132 mEq/L, Cl 105 mEq/L,
- Glucose: 295 mg/dl
- BUN: 48 mg/dl
- Creatinine: 1.1 mg/100 ml
- Urinalysis: pending
- Serum and urine myoglobin: pending
- Coagulation profile: normal

Radiographs

- Chest x-ray: no gross pathology
- Abdominal x-ray: no gross pathology

Questions

Read each question carefully, keeping in mind the context of the case under discussion. Select the best answer from the choices presented.

1. Your patient is one of approximately how many people who suffer some form of thermal injury each year?
   A. 200
   B. 2,000
   C. 200,000
   D. 2,000,000

2. Your first two steps in treating a burn patient should involve
   A. Extinguishing any residual fire and obtaining a full set of vital signs
   B. Bandaging the burned areas and administering oxygen
   C. Extinguishing any residual fire and ensuring a patent airway
   D. Determining the percentage of body burns and ensuring a patent airway

3. Your assessment of the extent of your patient's burns indicates
   A. 15% to 25% first degree burns and 1% to 10% second degree burns
   B. 15% to 25% second degree burns and 15% to 25% third degree burns
   C. 25% to 35% second degree burns and 1% to 10% third degree burns
   D. 15% to 25% second degree burns and 1% to 10% third degree burns

4. Your initial evaluation of this patient's condition reveals total body surface burns of
   A. 1% to 10%
   B. 15% to 35%
   C. 40% to 50%
   D. An estimate of the total body surface burns cannot be made

5. Your patient is best classified as having sustained
   A. Major critical burns
   B. Moderate uncomplicated burns
   C. Minor burn injuries
   D. Flash burns

6. Which of the following basic life support field treatment modalities are appropriate for your patient?
   A. Administer humidified oxygen
   B. Cover burn areas with an antibacterial agent
   C. Cover burn areas with a sterile burn sheet
   D. Remove constricting items such as rings and bracelets if possible
   E. A, B, and D are correct
   F. A, D, and C are correct
   G. All of the above are correct
   H. None of the above are correct

7. The findings of buccal erythema, wheezing, and facial burns, and the possibility of noxious fumes should alert you to the possibility of
   A. Hematemesis
   B. Pleural effusion
   C. Rib fractures
   D. Airway obstruction or pulmonary edema

8. Your transportation time to the hospital is approximately 45 minutes. You should
   A. Attempt an IV with D5/W
   B. Attempt an IV with normal saline or Ringer's lactate
   C. Not attempt an IV because it increases the chance of infection
   D. Attempt an IV with packed red blood cells

9. Your patient's initial EKG shows
   A. Sinus rhythm with occasional unifocal PVCs
   B. Second degree heart block
   C. Sinus tachycardia with occasional unifocal PVCs
   D. Sinus rhythm with occasional multifocal PVCs

10. Which of the following late-stage complications might your patient be expected to develop in the hospital?
    A. Diabetes mellitus
    B. Infection
    C. Hyperalbuminemia
    D. Contractures
    E. A and D are correct
    F. B and D are correct
    G. A and C are correct
    H. None of the above are correct

11. Carboxyhemoglobin determinations are important in this case
    A. To determine if CO poisoning is present
    B. To estimate the extent of infection
    C. To determine the cause of the patient's low pCO2
    D. To accurately measure renal function

12. When you contact medical control, the physician advises you to initiate fluid replacement in accordance with the Parkland Burn Formula. Your IV administration set has a gtt/ml of 15. Based on this information, you should adjust your drip rate to be within the range of:
    A. 175 to 275 gtt/min
    B. 75 to 175 gtt/min
    C. 50 to 75 gtt/min
    D. 1 to 50 gtt/min

13. Acute renal insufficiency in hospitalized burn patients is often precipitated by all of the following except
    A. Myoglobinuria
    B. Burn shock
    C. Cardiogenic shock secondary to an anterior wall MI
    D. Coagulopathy

14. In your patient, which of the following respiratory emergencies must be watched for carefully?
    A. Tracheal collapse
    B. Acute emphysema
    C. Laryngeal or pulmonary edema
    D. Airway obstruction secondary to acute pneumothorax
    E. Hydrothorax

15. Looking at your patient's laboratory values (see "Laboratory Results"), you note the presence of leukocytosis and hyperglycemia. This finding
    A. Indicates massive infection
    B. Is definitive evidence that your patient is diabetic
    C. Is probably a laboratory error
    D. Is most likely the body's normal response to a massive traumatic injury

16. Two standard systems of calculating percentage body burns are
    A. The Rule of Nines chart and the Parkland Formula
    B. The Lund and Browder chart and the Rule of Nines chart
    C. The Evans and Baxter chart and the Rule of Nines chart
    D. The Cornell burn chart and the Rule of Nines chart

17. As an immediate intravenous replacement fluid
    A. D5/W is highly recommended because it provides the greatest increase in intravascular volume as well as being an energy source

B. Infusion of potassium-supplemented fluid is called for to correct the expected hypokalemia
C. Lactated Ringer's solution is contraindicated due to the patient's expected hyperkalemia
D. A packed red blood cell infusion should be set up immediately to combat anemia
E. D5/W is not the fluid of choice because it essentially supplies only free water, which does not remain within the intravascular space very long; a crystalloid solution is preferable

18. Infections in patients with extensive burns
    A. Are a common cause of later complications
    B. Are usually preventable with proper in-field precautions
    C. Can be prevented by in-field use of an antibacterial cream
    D. Usually present minimal problems due to the leukocytosis normally present
    E. A and C are correct
    F. B and D are correct
    G. A and B are correct

19. Your patient's initial vital signs are
    A. Strong evidence of an underlying hypertensive condition
    B. Indicative of a life-threatening arrhythmia
    C. Not uncommon for a patient such as yours
    D. Indicative of more than adequate hydration
    E. Most likely the result of a pulmonary embolism

Discussion

Your patient is one of approximately 2,000,000 people who suffer from some type of thermal injury each year in the United States. Of those burned, approximately 100,000 are hospitalized and some 12,000 die, many from late-stage massive infections. Organisms frequently involved include staphylococci and pseudomonas. Remember that necrotic tissue provides an excellent growth medium. Because burn patients often require extensive hospitalization, they are prone to a variety of complications, including pneumonia, contractures, and acute renal insufficiency. This latter condition may be precipitated by burn shock, coagulopathy, or myoglobinuria, the last of which has profound adverse effects upon the tubular systems of the kidney.

When you pull up to a fire scene, it is important to determine the nature of the fire and the approximate time that any victims spent trapped in it. With industrial fires, keep in mind the possibility of noxious fumes (chlorine, ammonia, nitrogen oxides, sulfur dioxide, and phosgene). Furthermore, confinement in enclosed areas (as experienced by your patient) for any extended time may complicate injuries from smoke inhalation. Since fires often result in high levels of carbon monoxide

(CO) in the surrounding air, check all burn victims, especially those who have been confined in enclosed spaces and those suffering loss of consciousness, for signs of CO poisoning. Classically, such poisoning results in cherry-red lips, but absence of this finding certainly does not rule out the possibility. Measurement of carboxyhemoglobin levels will indicate whether CO poisoning has occurred. Because CO has a hemoglobin-binding affinity 200 to 300 times as great as that of oxygen, affected persons become severely hypoxemic. Treatment consists of administering 100% oxygen or hyperbaric oxygen therapy, if available.

When you encounter a burn victim, your first steps should be to put out any remaining flames or smoldering clothing and, as in all cases, ensure a patent airway. Do not attempt further evaluation until both these steps have been properly managed. Following your primary survey, measure vital signs and perform a complete secondary survey.

Extensive burn injuries are one of the most traumatic insults the human body can suffer. Your patient's increased blood pressure and respiratory rate reflect the body's response to severe stress and pain. These are common findings for such a patient and result from a generalized "fight or flight" response characterized by massive sympathetic discharge. The hospital findings of leukocytosis and hyperglycemia at this early stage are probably due to the body's massive secretion of both steroids (*i.e.,* cortisol) and catecholamines (*i.e.,* epinephrine). Infection may also result in these elevated values, but is more likely to occur later in the patient's course.

Since a great percentage of burn patients die from respiratory involvement resulting from smoke and toxic fume inhalation, carefully examining your patient for signs of this complication is vital. Facial burns, singeing of facial hairs, swelling and redness of the buccal mucosa, wheezing, and the probability of noxious fumes should strongly suggest to you that your patient has suffered some type of inhalation injury. The possibility of your patient developing airway obstruction from laryngeal edema is certainly a dangerous one. Furthermore, the nature of the fire (noxious fumes and heavy smoke conditions) and the reported location of your patient (unconscious in a back room), along with your findings of wheezing and rhonchi, raise the possibility of impending pulmonary edema. Such edema may develop immediately or, in many cases, 24 to 48 hours after the initial injury. It is important to realize that pulmonary edema resulting from inhalation injuries is of noncardiac origin and demands different treatment modalities than would be used for pulmonary edema secondary to cardiac failure.

Since your secondary survey showed no gross abnormalities such as fractures or deformities or any other major injuries, your next step in patient evaluation involves calculating the extent and type of your patient's burns. Two standard techniques involve the Rule of Nines chart and the Lund and Browder chart. Both these charts divide the body into different regions and assign a specific percentage of the patient's total body surface area to each. Evaluating your patient's burns using the Lund and Browder chart (see Figure 13-3), we see that he has suffered the following percentage of body burns:

Burns on the entire face: 3.5%
Burns on the entire anterior trunk: 14%

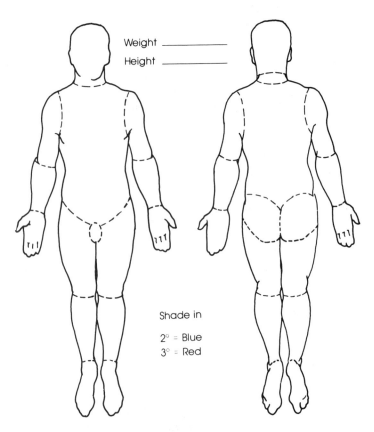

Area	Age — Years					% 2°	% 3°	% Total
	0-1	1-4	5-9	10-15	Adults			
Head	19	17	13	10	7			
Neck	2	2	2	2	2			
Ant. Trunk	13	17	13	13	13			
Post. Trunk	13	13	13	13	13			
R. Buttock	2½	2½	2½	2½	2½			
L. Buttock	2½	2½	2½	2½	2½			
Genitalia	1	1	1	1	1			
R. U. Arm	4	4	4	4	4			
L. U. Arm	4	4	4	4	4			
R. L. Arm	3	3	3	3	3			
L. L. Arm	3	3	3	3	3			
R. Hand	2½	2½	2½	2½	2½			
L. Hand	2½	2½	2½	2½	2½			
R. Thigh	5½	6½	8½	8½	9½			
L. Thigh	5½	6½	8½	8½	9½			
R. Leg	5	5	5½	6	7			
L. Leg	5	5	5½	6	7			
R. Foot	3½	3½	3½	3½	3½			
L. Foot	3½	3½	3½	3½	3½			
					Total			

FIGURE 13–3. Lund and Browder chart. (Hardy JD [ed]: Hardy's Textbook of Surgery, 2nd ed, p 178. Philadelphia, JB Lippincott, 1988)

Burns on the right palmar surface: 1.5%
Burns on the left palmar surface: 1.5%
Burns on the left anterior forearm: 1.5%
Total percentage body burns = 22%

The Rule of Nines chart, although less accurate, will give an answer of the same order of magnitude (Figure 13–4).

Burns are classically divided into three functionally significant types based on their depth of penetration. First degree burns involve only the most superficial layers of the skin and are characterized by redness but no blistering. Your patient showed no such burns. Second degree burns penetrate the entire epidermis and extend into parts of the underlying dermis. Such burns are characterized by erythema, blistering, and severe pain. This type of burn covers your patient's entire anterior trunk (14%) as well as his entire face (3.5%), yielding a total of approximately 17.5% second degree burns. Third degree burns involve the epidermis, the dermis, and also the underlying subcutaneous tissue. They are normally evidenced

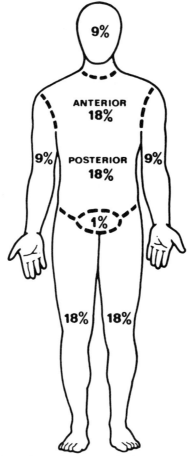

FIGURE 13–4. Rule of Nines chart. (Hardy JD (ed): Hardy's Textbook of Surgery, 2nd ed, p 177. Philadelphia, JB Lippincott, 1988)

by a charred or pearly-white appearance. Your patient shows this type of burn on the right palmar surface (1.5%), the left palmar surface (1.5%), and also along the entire anterior left forearm (1.5%), for a total of approximately 4.5% third degree burns.

The severity of a patient's burn injuries depends largely on the extent of the burns, the type of the burns, and the parts of the body involved. As a general rule, burns involving the hands, face, feet, genitalia, ears, and eyes, as well as all inhalation injuries, are considered major burn injuries. Your patient, suffering major burns on the face and hands as well as a probable inhalation injury, is classified as having sustained major burn injuries.

After completing your full evaluation, begin basic life support treatment, including administering humidified oxygen to combat hypoxemia, covering the burned areas with a sterile dressing or burn sheet to help prevent infection, and removing any rings and bracelets to prevent circulation cut-off should tissue edema develop. Do not use antibacterial agents in the field because they only make in-hospital cleansing and debridement more difficult.

Faced with a transportation time to the hospital of approximately 45 minutes, you should attempt to start an intravenous (IV) line. This serves two functions. First, and most importantly, it allows you to initiate fluid replacement to prevent large-scale fluid loss. Second, it provides a rapid access route should your patient require any medications. Your choice of an IV solution should be one such as normal saline or lactated Ringer's, both of which are crystalloid solutions. These solutions expand intravascular volume to a much greater extent than D5/W, which provides essentially only "free water" and does not remain within the intravascular space for any considerable period of time. Colloidal volume-expanding solutions such as human plasma protein fraction (Plasmanate) may also be used if available.

Having selected an IV solution, next determine the rate at which to maintain your IV drip. The Parkland Burn Formula is commonly used to estimate the necessary rate of initial fluid replacement. According to this formula:

$$\text{Total amount of lactated Ringer's solution to be infused over the first 8 hours after the burn} = \frac{\text{Patient's weight in kilograms} \times \text{The total percentage of body burns (all degrees)} \times 4.0 \text{ ml}}{2}$$

Since your patient weighs approximately 175 pounds (80 kg) and has total body surface burns of approximately 22%, the total amount of lactated Ringer's solution to be infused over the first 8 hours after the burn is roughly 3,520 ml. To calculate the initial drip rate, use the formula:

$$\text{gtt/min} = \frac{\text{Total volume of solution to be infused (ml)} \times \text{The gtt/ml of your administration set}}{\text{Total time over which fluid is to be infused (min)}}$$

Since your administration set delivers 15 drops per milliliter (gtt/ml = 15) and you wish to infuse a total volume of 3,520 ml over the first 8 hours (480 min), you should adjust your drip rate to deliver about 110 drops per minute (110 gtt/min).

> **Field Diagnosis**
> - Major burn injuries
> - Cardiac arrhythmia
>
> **Hospital Diagnosis**
> - Major burn injuries

Patient Follow-Up

Shortly after admission your patient developed progressively worsening respiratory distress, necessitating elective intubation and ventilatory support. After a prolonged hospital course complicated by renal failure and sepsis, your patient was finally discharged without any major sequela.

Answers

1. D

   Caroline NL: Emergency Care in the Streets, 3rd ed, p 380. Boston, Little, Brown & Co, 1987

   Caroline NL: Emergency Medical Treatment: A Text for EMT-As and EMT-Intermediates, 2nd ed, p 231. Boston, Little, Brown & Co, 1987

2. C

   American Academy of Orthopaedic Surgeons: Emergency Care and Transportation of the Sick and Injured, 4th ed, pp 415–416. Menasha, WI, George Banta Co, 1987

   Caroline NL: Emergency Medical Treatment: A Text for EMT-As and EMT-Intermediates, 2nd ed, pp 231–232. Boston, Little, Brown & Co, 1987

   Caroline NL: Emergency Care in the Streets, 3rd ed, p 384. Boston, Little, Brown & Co, 1987

3. D

   American Academy of Orthopaedic Surgeons: Emergency Care and Transportation of the Sick and Injured, 4th ed, pp 414–415. Menasha, WI, George Banta Co, 1987

   Grant HD, Murray RH Jr, Bergeron JD: Emergency Care, 4th ed, p 409. Englewood Cliffs, NJ, Prentice-Hall, 1986

   Caroline NL: Emergency Care in the Streets, 3rd ed, p 383. Boston, Little, Brown & Co, 1987

4. B

   Caroline NL: Emergency Medical Treatment: A Text for EMT-As and EMT-Intermediates, 2nd ed, pp 233–234. Boston, Little, Brown & Co, 1987

   Grant HD, Murray RH Jr, Bergeron JD: Emergency Care, 4th ed, p 409. Englewood Cliffs, NJ, Prentice-Hall, 1986

   Caroline NL: Emergency Care in the Streets, 3rd ed, p 383. Boston, Little, Brown & Co, 1987

5. A

   Caroline NL: Emergency Care in the Streets, 3rd ed, p 382. Boston, Little, Brown & Co, 1987

   Caroline NL: Emergency Medical Treatment: A Text for EMT-As and EMT-Intermediates, 2nd ed, p 234. Boston, Little, Brown & Co, 1987

   Grant HD, Murray RH Jr, Bergeron JD: Emergency Care, 4th ed, p 410. Englewood Cliffs, NJ, Prentice-Hall, 1986

6. **F**

American Academy of Orthopaedic Surgeons: Emergency Care and Transportation of the Sick and Injured, 4th ed, pp 415–416. Menasha, WI, George Banta Co, 1987

Caroline NL: Emergency Medical Treatment: A Text for EMT-As and EMT-Intermediates, 2nd ed, pp 234–236. Boston, Little, Brown & Co, 1987

Caroline NL: Emergency Care in the Streets, 3rd ed, pp 283–285. Boston, Little, Brown & Co, 1987

7. **D**

Caroline NL: Emergency Care in the Streets, 3rd ed, p 384. Boston, Little, Brown & Co, 1987

Caroline NL: Emergency Medical Treatment: A Text for EMT-As and EMT-Intermediates, 2nd ed, p 232. Boston, Little, Brown & Co, 1987

8. **B**

Caroline NL: Emergency Care in the Streets, 3rd ed, p 385. Boston, Little, Brown & Co, 1987

Caroline NL: Emergency Medical Treatment: A Text for EMT-As and EMT-Intermediates, 2nd ed, p 232. Boston, Little, Brown & Co, 1987

9. **A**

Huff J, Doernbach DP, White RD: ECG Workout: Exercises in Arrhythmia Interpretation, pp 144, 242. Philadelphia, JB Lippincott, 1985

10. **F**

Pruitt BA Jr, Goodwin CW Jr: Burns: Including cold, chemical, and electrical injuries. In Sabiston DC Jr (ed): Textbook of Surgery, 13th ed. Philadelphia, WB Saunders, 1986

11. **A**

Caroline NL: Emergency Medical Treatment: A Text for EMT-As and EMT-Intermediates, 2nd ed, pp 425–426. Boston, Little, Brown & Co, 1987

Caroline NL: Emergency Care in the Streets, 3rd ed, pp 449–450. Boston, Little, Brown & Co, 1987

Bronston PK, Corre KA, Decker SJ: Carbon monoxide poisoning: A review. Top Emerg Med 8:50, 1987

12. **B**

Pruitt BA Jr, Goodwin CW Jr: Burns: Including cold, chemical, and electrical injuries. In Sabiston DC Jr (ed): Textbook of Surgery, 13th ed, pp 218–219. Philadelphia, WB Saunders, 1986

13. **C**

Pruitt BA Jr, Goodwin CW Jr: Burns: Including cold, chemical, and electrical injuries. In Sabiston DC Jr (ed): Textbook of Surgery, 13th ed. Philadelphia, WB Saunders, 1986

14. **C**

Caroline NL: Emergency Medical Treatment: A Text for EMT-As and EMT-Intermediates, 2nd ed, p 232. Boston, Little, Brown & Co, 1987

Caroline NL: Emergency Care in the Streets, 3rd ed, pp 284–286. Boston, Little, Brown & Co, 1987

15. **D**

Pruitt BA Jr, Goodwin CW Jr: Burns: Including cold, chemical, and electrical injuries. In Sabiston DC Jr (ed): Textbook of Surgery, 13th ed. Philadelphia, WB Saunders, 1986

16. **B**

Caroline NL: Emergency Care in the Streets, 3rd ed, pp 382–383. Boston, Little, Brown & Co, 1987

Caroline NL: Emergency Medical Treatment: A Text for EMT-As and EMT-Intermediates, 2nd ed, pp 233–234. Boston, Little, Brown & Co, 1987

Forstater AT (ed): Emergency Medicine Reference Book, pp 68–69. New York, Pfizer Laboratories, 1981

17. **E**

Caroline NL: Emergency Medical Treatment: A Text for EMT-As and EMT-Intermediates, 2nd ed, p 232. Boston, Little, Brown & Co, 1987

Caroline NL: Emergency Care in the Streets, 3rd ed, pp 74–76, 385. Boston, Little, Brown & Co, 1987

18. **A**

Pruitt BA Jr, Goodwin CW Jr: Burns: Including cold, chemical, and electrical injuries. In Sabiston DC Jr (ed): Textbook of Surgery, 13th ed. Philadelphia, WB Saunders, 1986

19. **C**

Pruitt BA Jr, Goodwin CW Jr: Burns: Including cold, chemical, and electrical injuries. In Sabiston DC Jr (ed): Textbook of Surgery, 13th ed. Philadelphia, WB Saunders, 1986

Selected Reading

Bronston PK, Corre KA, Decker SJ: Carbon monoxide poisoning: a review. Top Emerg Med 8:50, 1987

Frank HA, Wachtel TL (eds): Thermal injuries. Top Emerg Med 3:3, 1981

Goodwin CW, Dorothy J, Lam V, Pruitt BA, Jr.: Randomized trial of efficiency of crystalloid and colloid resuscitation on hemodynamic response and lung water following thermal injury. Ann Surg 197:520, 1983

Jelenko C III, Matthews JB: Burns and electrical injuries. In Tintinalli JE, Rothstein RJ, Krome RL (eds): Emergency Medicine: A Comprehensive Study Guide. New York, McGraw-Hill 1985

Moncrief JA: Burns. N Engl J Med 288:444, 1973

Pruitt BA Jr, Goodwin CW Jr: Burns: Including cold, chemical, and electrical injuries. In Sabiston DC Jr (ed): Textbook of Surgery, 13th ed. Philadelphia, WB Saunders, 1986

Shuck JM, Moncrie JA: Burns: Thermal, electrical, and chemical injuries. In Schwartz GR, Safar P, Stone JH, Storey PB, Wagner DK (eds): Principles and Practice of Emergency Medicine, 2nd ed. Philadelphia, WB Saunders, 1986

14

Thoracoabdominal Pain Following a Fall

Your ambulance responds to a call involving a young man with "abdominal pains." After securing your vehicle in front of a two-family private house, you are greeted by a middle-aged man who tells you that his son fell off a ladder while painting and hurt his stomach.

As you enter the house, you find the patient lying on the sofa in a right lateral recumbent position, with both knees drawn up to his chest. The parents tell you that about 2 to 3 hours ago, their son fell 8 to 10 feet off a ladder while he was painting the side of the house. Further questioning indicates that the patient landed on his left side, and although he did not lose consciousness, he did require assistance into the house.

Your patient is a 24-year-old man weighing approximately 180 pounds. He is conscious, alert, and oriented. He appears to be in moderate distress and complains of intense pain "on the left side." The pain, he says, started immediately after he fell from the ladder. He describes it as "sharp and intense" and says it is aggravated by movement, coughing, or deep breathing. It is localized over the lower left rib cage, upper left abdominal quadrant, and also over the left flank. Questioning reveals no loss of consciousness or vomiting.

The patient's medical history indicates a preexisting asthma condition and an appendectomy at the age of 19. You are also told that he has a heart murmur that is "not serious" and that has been present since childhood. No history of rheumatic fever is reported. Medications include isoetharine hydrochloride (Bronkosol) and an over-the-counter vitamin supplement. No allergies are reported.

Upon your arrival, vital signs measured with the patient in a supine position are BP 116/78 (right arm, by auscultation), pulse 98 and regular, and respiration 32 regular and shallow. Orthostatic vital signs measured with the patient elevated at a 45 degree angle are BP 106/68 (right arm, by auscultation), pulse 112 and regular, and respiration 29 regular and shallow.

Physical examination indicates no signs of trauma or injury to the head or neck. The trachea appears midline, and no surrounding signs of deformity or soft tissue injury are noted. Cervical spine point tenderness is absent, and no paravertebral muscle spasms are felt.

Examination of the ears, eyes, nose and throat is unremarkable. No postauricular ecchymosis is found. Blood and cerebrospinal fluid appear absent from the ears and nose. The mouth is clear of blood, vomit and other foreign matter.

Observation of the thorax reveals bruising over the lower left lateral portion of the rib cage. Respiratory excursion appears unilaterally diminished on the left side. Palpation indicates marked tenderness over the left seventh and eighth ribs, as well as along the costal margin on the left side. Auscultation reveals normal vesicular and bronchovesicular sounds bilaterally. No rhonchi or rales are appreciated. Heart sounds are clear and crisp with normal S_1S_2. The point of maximal impulse is located in the fifth intercostal space, just medial to the midclavicular line.

Abdominal examination shows a yellowish blue discoloration around the umbilicus and an old scar in the lower right quadrant. Auscultation for 2 minutes reveals no bowel sounds. Palpation demonstrates general rigidity and marked tenderness in the upper left abdominal quadrant. Tenderness is also noted over the left flank and radiates around to the back.

Neurologic examination demonstrates an alert and oriented individual. Pupils are round, equal and reactive to light. No tenderness is noted along the vertebral column. Movement and sensation are present in all four extremities and the patient has no complaints of paresis or paresthesia. No evidence of deformity is found in the extremities or in the pelvic girdle, and the remainder of the examination is normal.

The patient is placed on an EKG monitor and a lead II six-second strip is recorded (Figure 14–1). You contact medical control and begin appropriate field treatment. Vital signs repeated with the patient in a supine position are BP 88/60 (right arm, by auscultation), pulse 152 and irregular, and respiration 16 regular and shallow. During transport to the hospital, you continue to monitor vital signs at 5-minute intervals and to carry out continuous cardiac monitoring.

Questions

Read each question carefully, keeping in mind the context of the case under discussion. Select the best answer from the choices presented.

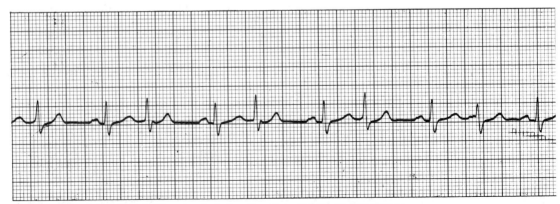

FIGURE 14–1. Lead II EKG recorded shortly after arrival at the scene.

1. Retroperitoneal structures include the
   1. Kidneys
   2. Liver
   3. Adrenal glands
   4. Stomach

   A. 1, 2, and 3 are correct
   B. 1 and 3 are correct
   C. 2 and 4 are correct
   D. Only 4 is correct
   E. All are correct

2. Which of the following are considered "hollow" organs?
   1. Stomach
   2. Large intestine
   3. Gallbladder
   4. Urinary bladder

   A. 1, 2, and 3 are correct
   B. 1 and 3 are correct
   C. 2 and 4 are correct
   D. Only 4 is correct
   E. All are correct

3. Which of the following are classified as "solid" organs?
   1. Liver
   2. Adrenal glands
   3. Spleen
   4. Pancreas

   A. 1, 2, and 3 are correct
   B. 1 and 3 are correct
   C. 2 and 4 are correct
   D. Only 4 is correct
   E. All are correct

4. The patient's complaint of left-sided thoracoabdominal pain that is aggravated by movement, coughing, or deep breathing suggests
   A. Acute pulmonary embolism
   B. Rib fracture
   C. Acute myocardial infarction
   D. Ruptured aortic aneurysm

5. The initial vital signs taken upon arrival suggest
   A. Normal intravascular volume
   B. Decreased intravascular volume
   C. Increased intravascular volume
   D. None of the above

6. The patient's initial EKG (Figure 14-1) contains which of the following?
    1. Normal sinus beats
    2. Junctional beats
    3. Premature atrial beats
    4. Agonal idioventricular beats

    A. 1, 2, and 3 are correct
    B. 1 and 3 are correct
    C. 2 and 4 are correct
    D. Only 4 is correct
    E. All are correct

7. Treatment of this patient is best based on the field diagnosis of
    1. Rib fracture
    2. Possible spinal injury
    3. Intraabdominal bleeding
    4. Ruptured spleen

    A. 1, 2, and 3 are correct
    B. 1 and 3 are correct
    C. 2 and 4 are correct
    D. Only 4 is correct
    E. All are correct

8. Treatment of this patient calls for
    1. Administering oxygen
    2. Applying MAST
    3. Establishing a large bore intravenous line
    4. Rapid transport

    A. 1, 2, and 3 are correct
    B. 1 and 3 are correct
    C. 2 and 4 are correct
    D. Only 4 is correct
    E. All are correct

9. The most commonly injured organ in cases of blunt abdominal trauma is the
    A. Liver
    B. Colon
    C. Appendix
    D. Spleen

Discussion

Traumatic abdominal injuries fall into two broad categories. *Open* injuries are those in which a foreign object has penetrated the abdominal cavity (*e.g.,* a bullet or knife). *Closed* injuries are those in which the abdominal contents are injured as a result of a forceful blow. Such *blunt trauma* most often occurs as a result of a physical assault, a motor vehicle accident or, as in this case, a fall. Although all the organs in the abdominal cavity are subject to injury from blunt trauma, the size, location and fragility of the spleen make it the solid organ most frequently injured in cases of blunt abdominal trauma.

The abdominal cavity lies below the thoracic cavity and is bound inferiorly by an imaginary plane running from the pubis to the sacrum, superiorly by the diaphragm, and anteriorly and posteriorly by the peritoneum and the associated musculoskeletal wall. For purposes of localization and description, the external anterior surface of the abdominal (or abdominopelvic) cavity may be divided into four quadrants or nine regions (Figures 14-2 and 14-3). The upper left abdominal quadrant, for instance, contains the spleen, stomach, and portions of the colon, while the appendix is found in the lower right abdominal quadrant.

Taken in total, the findings of diminished respiratory excursion, bruising over the rib cage, tenderness over the seventh and eighth ribs, and abdominal tenderness and rigidity in your patient strongly suggest both rib fracture(s) and blunt abdominal trauma. The location of the pain along the left flank, and the fact that it radiates to the back, suggest injury to the underlying kidney, rather than to the liver, gallbladder or appendix, all of which are located on the right side of the body. Pain in the upper left quadrant strongly suggests the possibility of a damaged or ruptured spleen (the most commonly injured solid organ in the abdominal cavity). Three factors strongly suggest major internal bleeding: orthostatic changes in vital signs, Cullen's sign and abdominal rigidity. *Orthostatic changes* are measured changes in blood pressure and pulse rate that result when the patient is shifted from a supine to a sitting position. In cases where circulating blood volume is significantly decreased

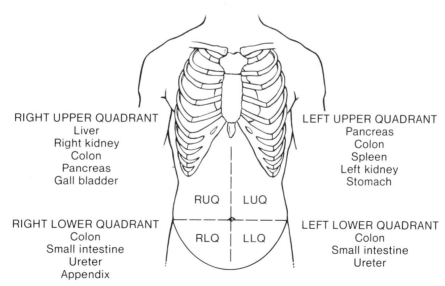

FIGURE 14-2. Division of abdominopelvic cavity into four quadrants showing organ contents of each quadrant. (Greenberg MD, Lieber JJ: Abdominal trauma. J Emerg Care Transport 13(2):86, 1984)

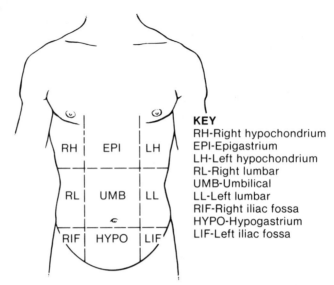

FIGURE 14-3. Division of abdominopelvic cavity into nine regions using two transverse and two horizontal planes. (Greenberg MD, Lieber JJ: Abdominal trauma. J Emerg Care Transport 13(2):86, 1984)

(hypovolemia), a fall in blood pressure and an increase in pulse rate (compensative tachycardia) occur. These changes reflect the body's unsuccessful attempt to maintain cardiac output in the face of increased demands. *Cullen's sign* is a yellowish blue discoloration that may be found around the umbilicus in cases of intraperitoneal or retroperitoneal hemorrhage. *Abdominal rigidity* results when irritative stimuli (blood, gastric contents, ruptured appendix, etc.) cause reflexive spasms of the abdominal musculature. While not pathognomonic of internal bleeding in this clinical setting, such rigidity does strongly suggest it.

Treatment should be oriented toward correcting the deteriorating cardiovascular function and preventing shock. Administer high-flow/high-concentration oxygen to correct any underlying hypoxemia. Place the patient in a supine position to promote venous return, apply military antishock trousers (MAST), and inflate them if local protocols and the patient's blood pressure require. Establish at least one large bore intravenous (IV) line and administer a volume replacement fluid such as Ringer's lactate. Constantly monitor vital signs and cardiac function. Because definitive treatment can only be provided in the hospital, rapid transport is important.

Field Diagnosis

- Intraabdominal hemorrhage
- Ruptured spleen
- Fractured rib(s), left chest
- Spinal injury
- Cardiac arrhythmia

(Continued)

> **Hospital Diagnosis** *(Continued)*
> - Intraabdominal hemorrhage secondary to splenic rupture
> - Fracture involving left eighth, ninth, and tenth ribs
> - Cardiac arrhythmia, etiology unknown

Patient Follow-Up

Following admission to the hospital your patient continued to demonstrate increasing abdominal rigidity and serious hemodynamic instability. A stat chest radiograph demonstrated fractures involving the eighth, ninth, and tenth ribs of the left side of the chest (Figure 14–4). A laparotomy revealed splenic rupture with significant blood loss. Following aggressive surgical treatment your patient underwent an uncomplicated postoperative course and was discharged from the hospital.

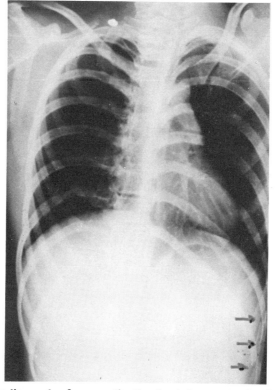

FIGURE 14–4. Radiograph of your patient's chest demonstrating fractures of the left eighth, ninth, and tenth ribs. (Cosgriff JH Jr, Anderson DL: The Practice of Emergency Care, 2nd ed, p 371. Philadelphia, JB Lippincott, 1984)

Answers

1. B
   Caroline NL: Emergency Medical Treatment: A Text for EMT-As and EMT-Intermediates, 2nd ed, p 300. Boston, Little, Brown & Co, 1987

2. E
   Caroline NL: Emergency Medical Treatment: A Text for EMT-As and EMT-Intermediates, 2nd ed, p 301. Boston, Little, Brown & Co, 1987

3. E
   Caroline NL: Emergency Medical Treatment: A Text for EMT-As and EMT-Intermediates, 2nd ed, p 301. Boston, Little, Brown & Co, 1987

4. B
   Caroline NL: Emergency Care in the Streets, 3rd ed, pp 201–202. Boston, Little, Brown & Co, 1987

5. B
   Caroline NL: Emergency Care in the Streets, 3rd ed, pp 78–80. Boston, Little, Brown & Co, 1987

6. A
   Huff J, Doernbach DP, White RD: ECG Workout: Exercises in Arrhythmia Interpretation, pp 112, 235 (strip 3.99). Philadelphia, JB Lippincott, 1985

7. E
   Caroline NL: Emergency Care in the Streets, 3rd ed, pp 78–80, 201, 356, 397–399. Boston, Little, Brown & Co, 1987

8. E
   Caroline NL: Emergency Medical Treatment: A Text for EMT-As and EMT-Intermediates, 2nd ed, pp 305–306. Boston, Little, Brown & Co, 1987
   Caroline NL: Emergency Care in the Streets, 3rd ed, p 398. Boston, Little, Brown & Co, 1987

9. D
   Krome RL: Abdominal trauma. In Tintinalli JE, Rothstein RJ, Krome RL (eds): Emergency Medicine: A Comprehensive Study Guide. New York, McGraw-Hill, 1985

Selected Reading

Bietz DS: Abdominal injuries. Emergency 10:30, 1978

Cosgriff JH Jr, Anderson DL: Thoracic and abdominal injuries. In Cosgriff JH Jr, Anderson DL: The Practice of Emergency Care, 2nd ed. Philadelphia, JB Lippincott, 1984

Hale HW Jr et al: Symposium on blunt abdominal trauma. Contemp Surg 10:39, 1977

Krome RL: Abdominal trauma. In Tintinalli JE, Rothstein RJ, Krome RL (eds): Emergency Medicine: A Comprehensive Study Guide. New York, McGraw-Hill, 1985

ADVANCED CARDIAC LIFE SUPPORT EMERGENCIES

15

Palpitations and Dyspnea

Your patient is a 48-year-old man who is complaining of a "funny" feeling in his chest. He reports feeling fine until approximately half an hour ago when he started to feel somewhat fatigued and developed this symptom. He has no significant past medical history, takes no medications, and reports no allergies. His vital signs are BP 98/78, pulse 150 and regular, and respiration 18 and regular. After initiating cardiac monitoring you see the following (Figure 15-1):

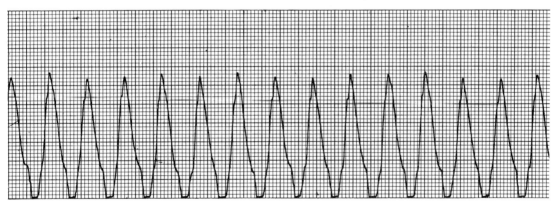

FIGURE 15-1

1. The patient's initial cardiac tracing (Figure 15-1) is most consistent with
   A. Ventricular fibrillation
   B. Sinus tachycardia
   C. Complete third degree AV block
   D. Ventricular tachycardia

A1: Inspection of the EKG (Figure 15-1) reveals a wide complex tachyarrhythmia at a rate of approximately 150 complexes per minute. The rhythm is regular, P waves are not seen, and the QRS complexes are wide and bizarre. This is most consistent with an interpretation of ventricular tachycardia (although a definite diagnosis is difficult to make with only a monitor lead EKG).

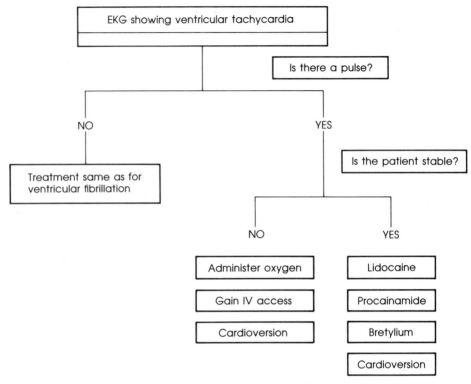

FIGURE 15-2. Management of ventricular tachycardia.

2. Initial treatment should consist of
   A. Lidocaine, 1 mg/kg bolus, followed by a drip
   B. Unsynchronized cardioversion, 100 Joules
   C. Atropine sulfate, 0.5 mg IV bolus
   D. Epinephrine, 1:10,000, 0.5 to 1.0 mg IV push

A2: Initial treatment of ventricular tachycardia depends on the presence or absence of a pulse and on the clinical state of the patient (Figure 15-2). When there is an associated pulse, treatment is dictated by the patient's condition. If the patient is judged to be hemodynamically stable (i.e., he has no chest pain, dyspnea, or hypotension, and has a systolic BP > 90 mm Hg), then, after establishing an intravenous (IV) line, attempt treatment with antiarrhythmic medications. The first line drug of choice is lidocaine, 1 mg/kg IV bolus, followed by an infusion at 2 mg/min. If ventricular tachycardia persists, continue to administer boluses of lidocaine, 0.5 mg/kg, at 8-minute intervals until either ventricular tachycardia resolves or a total dose of 3 mg/kg has been administered.

At this point your patient starts to complain of severe chest pain. Repeat vital signs show BP 82/64, pulse 188 and regular, and respiration 14 and regular. Cardiac monitoring reveals the following (Figure 15-3):

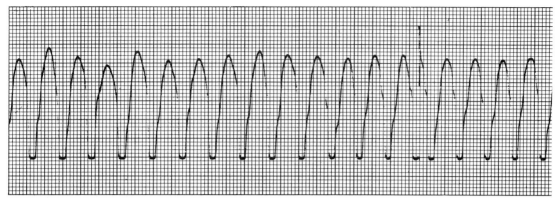

FIGURE 15-3

3. Treatment at this point should consist of
   A. Immediate cardioversion
   B. Procainamide, 20 mg/min IV infusion
   C. Lidocaine, 0.5 mg/kg IV bolus
   D. Epinephrine 1:10,000, 0.5 to 1.0 mg IV bolus

A3: Review of your patient's cardiac rhythm (Figure 15-3) reveals a rapid ventricular tachycardia associated with marked hypotension and clinical symptoms (*i.e.,* chest pain). Hemodynamically unstable ventricular tachycardia associated with a pulse calls for immediate corrective measures. The best approach is cardioversion, starting with 50 to 100 Joules (Figure 15-4).

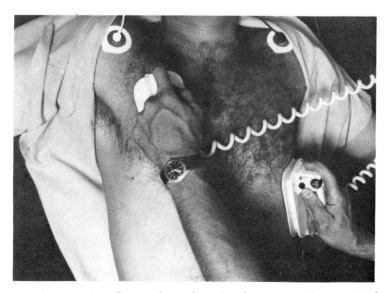

FIGURE 15-4. Procedure for cardioversion showing proper placement of paddles. (Blake-Bunting L, Parker J, Weigel A: Defibrillation: A Manual for the EMT, p 93. Philadelphia, JB Lippincott, 1985)

Following your initial cardioversion, your patient appears clinically improved: his chest pain has decreased and his blood pressure is 110/78. Cardiac monitoring at this point reveals the following (Figure 15-5):

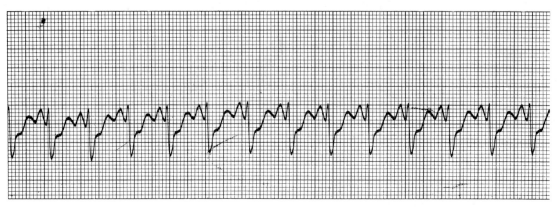

FIGURE 15-5

4. Your patient's cardiac rhythm (Figure 15-5) now demonstrates
   A. Sinus bradycardia
   B. Second degree AV heart block
   C. Atrial flutter
   D. Sinus tachycardia

A4: This tracing (Figure 15-5) reveals a regular rhythm at a rate of approximately 135 beats per minute. Each QRS complex is preceded by a discrete atrial P wave. This configuration reflects a sinus rhythm. Also notable in this tracing are the significant ST depression and large P waves. In summary, the patient's cardiac rhythm represents sinus tachycardia.

Further treatment should involve continued cardiac monitoring, frequent assessment of vital signs, and continued administration of a lidocaine infusion and supplemental oxygen.

Field Diagnosis
- Multiple cardiac arrhythmias

Hospital Diagnosis
- Acute myocardial infarction complicated by cardiac arrhythmias

Patient Follow-Up

Your patient was admitted to the coronary care unit for observation and treatment. Serial electrocardiograms and cardiac enzyme measurements confirmed the occurrence of a massive anterior wall myocardial infarction. On his second day in the hospital, the patient developed intractable malignant ventricular arrhythmias. Despite aggressive resuscitative measures, he died.

Answers

1. D
   Caroline NL: Emergency Care in the Streets, 3rd ed, p 299. Boston, Little, Brown & Co, 1987
   Huff J, Doernbach DP, White RD: ECG Workout: Exercises in Arrhythmia Interpretation, pp 142, 242 (strip 4.74). Philadelphia, JB Lippincott, 1985

2. A
   Caroline NL: Emergency Care in the Streets, 3rd ed, p 299. Boston, Little, Brown & Co, 1987
   Grauer K, Cavallaro D: ACLS: Certification Preparation and a Comprehensive Review, 2nd ed, pp 10-12. St Louis, CV Mosby, 1987
   American Heart Association: Standards and guidelines for cardiopulmonary resuscitation (CPR) and emergency cardiac care (ECC). JAMA 255:2905 (see pages 2946-2948), 1986

3. A
   Caroline NL: Emergency Care in the Streets, 3rd ed, p 333. Boston, Little, Brown & Co, 1987
   Grauer K, Cavallaro D: ACLS: Certification Preparation and a Comprehensive Review, 2nd ed, pp 10-12, 44-45. St Louis, CV Mosby, 1987
   American Heart Association: Standards and guidelines for cardiopulmonary resuscitation (CPR) and emergency cardiac care (ECC). JAMA 255:2905 (see pages 2946-2947), 1986

4. D
   Huff J, Doernbach DP, White RD: ECG Workout: Exercises in Arrhythmia Interpretation, pp 32, 217 (strip 1.79). Philadelphia, JB Lippincott, 1985

Selected Reading

American Heart Association: Standards and guidelines for cardiopulmonary resuscitation (CPR) and emergency cardiac care (ECC). JAMA 255:2905, 1986

16

Hypotension and an Altered Mental State in an Elderly Woman

Your ambulance responds to a report of a "woman down." After a short response interval, you pull up in front of a large department store. On the sidewalk surrounded by a group of onlookers, an elderly woman is lying face-up on the ground. You quickly gather your equipment and begin to assess the patient's condition. She responds to verbal stimuli but is lethargic and has difficulty answering questions. Primary survey shows that pulse and spontaneous respirations are present. There are no signs of major blood loss, and her cervical spine appears intact.

Vital signs on arrival are BP (right arm, supine) 80/70, pulse 40 weak and regular, and respirations 14 and regular. A quick physical examination reveals no signs of trauma. The pupils are round, equal, and reactive to light. The oropharynx is clear of foreign debris, vomitus, and blood. The trachea is midline. Heart sounds are not muffled and the lungs are clear to auscultation. No gross abdominal distension or injury is evident and spontaneous movement is present in all extremities. Cardiac monitoring reveals the following (Figure 16-1):

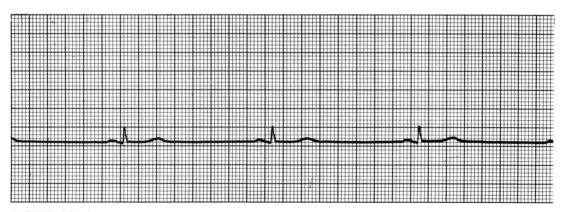

FIGURE 16-1

After instituting basic life support, you administer an intravenous medication and prepare your patient for transport. Vital signs repeated 5 minutes after arrival are BP 110/78, pulse 65, and respirations 14 and regular. Your patient is now alert and oriented to time, place, and self, and is able to answer questions coherently. A repeat EKG shows the following (Figure 16–2):

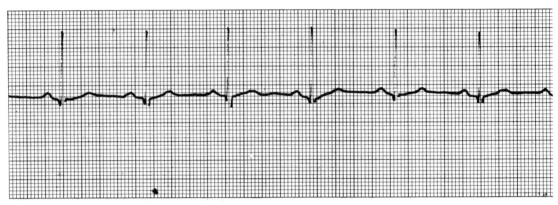

FIGURE 16-2

Questions

Read each question carefully, keeping in mind the context of the case under discussion. Select the best answer from the choices presented.

1. Initial treatment of this patient should include
    1. Administering supplemental oxygen
    2. Establishing an intravenous line
    3. Continuous cardiac monitoring
    4. Inflating MAST

    A. 1, 2, and 3 are correct
    B. 1 and 3 are correct
    C. 2 and 4 are correct
    D. Only 4 is correct
    E. All are correct

2. The patient's initial EKG (Figure 16–1) is characterized by all of the following except
    A. P waves of sinus origin
    B. QRS complexes of normal duration and morphology
    C. Normal PR interval
    D. An irregular rhythm

3. The patient's initial EKG (Figure 16-1) is best classified as
   A. Normal sinus rhythm
   B. Sinus arrhythmia
   C. Sinus bradycardia
   D. Complete third degree AV block
   E. A slow idioventricular escape rhythm

4. Appropriate medications in this case would include
   1. Calcium chloride, 10 ml, IV bolus
   2. Lidocaine, 100 mg, IV bolus
   3. Epinephrine, 0.5 mg, IV push
   4. Atropine, 0.5 mg, IV push

   A. 1, 2, and 3 are correct
   B. 1 and 3 are correct
   C. 2 and 4 are correct
   D. Only 4 is correct
   E. All are correct

5. Your patient's repeat EKG following administration of medication (Figure 16-2) is best classified as
   A. Normal sinus rhythm
   B. Sinus bradycardia
   C. Second degree AV block
   D. Sinus tachycardia
   E. Sinus arrhythmia

6. Based on your patient's second EKG (Figure 16-2), further medical treatment is best carried out with
   A. Lidocaine, 4 mg/min infusion
   B. A repeat dose of atropine, 0.5 to 1.0 mg, IV push
   C. An additional bolus of calcium chloride
   D. No further administration of medications

Discussion

In the present case, an elderly woman presents with an acutely altered mental state manifested by collapse, confusion, and lethargy. Significant findings during initial assessment include hypotension and bradycardia. There are no signs of gross trauma and the remainder of the physical examination contributes little to an etiologic diagnosis.

The patient's initial cardiac rhythm (Figure 16-1) is somewhat more useful in this case. Analysis of this strip reveals a regular rhythm at an atrial rate and a ventricular rate of 38 complexes per minute. P waves are present and upright, of uniform configuration, and precede each QRS complex, indicating that the rhythm is of sinus origin. The PR interval is constant and of normal duration at 0.14 to 0.16 seconds, indicating that no first degree AV block is present. Each QRS complex is preceded by a P wave, has a normal morphology, and is of normal duration (0.06 sec). A correct interpretation of this rhythm is sinus bradycardia at a rate of 38 complexes per minute.

Sinus bradycardia defines a sinus rhythm with a rate less than 60 complexes per minute (see "Electrocardiographic Characteristics of Sinus Bradycardia"). The

---

Electrocardiographic Characteristics of Sinus Bradycardia

P Waves

- Normal duration and morphology
- Upright in leads I, II, and aVF
- All have uniform configuration
- All are followed by a QRS complex

PR Interval

- Normal duration less than 0.21 sec (in an adult)

QRS Complex

- Normal duration and morphology
- Each complex is preceded by a P wave

ST Segment

- Without elevation or depression

T Wave

- Without abnormality

Rate

- Atrial and ventricular rate are identical and less than 60 per min, most frequently between 40 and 60 although it may be slower

Rhythm

- Regular atrial and ventricular rhythm is present
- In some cases slight irregularity in the rhythm may be present (*e.g.,* coexisting sinus arrhythmia)

Pacemaker

- SA node

Summary

A regular rhythm of sinus origin in which the SA node paces the heart at a rate of less than 60 beats per minute

---

P waves are of normal morphology and duration, indicating that the pacemaker is the SA node. The PR interval, QRS complexes, ST segment, and T waves are all normal. The major abnormality is simply a slow-firing SA node. Sinus bradycardia

TABLE 16-1. Etiology of Sinus Bradycardia

Physiologic	Medications	Medical Conditions
Sleep	Morphine	Acute myocardial infarction
Athletic conditioning	Propranolol	Chronic ischemic heart disease
Vagal maneuvers	Digitalis	Sinus node disease
	Reserpine	Hypothyroidism
	Clonidine	Increased intracranial pressure
		Hypothermia
		Alkalosis

occurs in a wide variety of settings; increased vagal tone, medications, and cardiac disease are a few of the causes (Table 16-1).

Clinically, the effects of sinus bradycardia largely depend on the underlying etiology, the health of the person, and the degree of bradycardia. Adverse hemodynamic effects are more common when the rate becomes excessively slow (*i.e.,* less than 40 complexes per minute) or when underlying cardiac disease results in diminished cardiac reserve. Since cardiac output is determined by the product of stroke volume and heart rate, an excessively slow heart rate may severely limit cardiac output, especially if cardiac reserve is minimal and the patient is unable to compensate by increasing stroke volume. In such cases the clinical picture may be characterized by signs of acute hemodynamic compromise, including:

- Light-headedness
- Dizziness
- Syncope
- Altered mental state
- Hypotension

Although the patient's presenting signs of syncope (or near-syncope), altered mentation, and hypotension may reflect a variety of conditions, their acute onset in association with an extremely slow sinus bradycardia at a rate of 38 complexes per minute strongly suggests that cardiac arrhythmia is the culprit. While no definitive determination can be made (in the field) about the cause of the arrhythmia, this practical and useful field diagnosis can guide further treatment.

Initial management of this patient should include measures such as establishing an intravenous (IV) line, administering supplemental oxygen, frequently monitoring vital signs, and constant cardiac monitoring. Two important questions arise: what is the specific treatment of sinus bradycardia and when is specific treatment required (Figure 16-3)? In a patient with EKG-documented sinus bradycardia the answer to the question—Is specific treatment required?—depends on whether the patient is symptomatic. If the sinus bradycardia is associated with clinical symptoms such as hypotension, ventricular escape beats, altered mentation, and chest pain, then specific treatment is warranted. On the other hand, if there are minimal or no adverse signs or symptoms, then no specific treatment is warranted and basic supportive measures and transport to a medical facility for further workup will suffice. This patient's documented sinus bradycardia is associated with significant

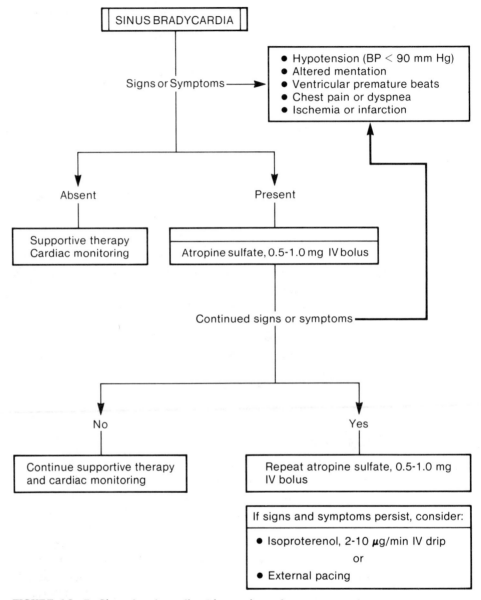

FIGURE 16-3. Sinus bradycardia: Diagnosis and management.

clinical symptoms, including hypotension and altered mentation. Specific treatment is therefore required.

The specific medical treatment of clinically symptomatic sinus bradycardia includes the initial administration of atropine sulfate. Atropine sulfate is an anticholinergic agent with parasympatholytic effects (see "Atropine Sulfate"). It inhibits vagal impulses in the heart, resulting in enhanced AV conduction and an

Atropine Sulfate

Class

Parasympatholytic agent

Historical Perspective

Atropine sulfate is a naturally occurring compound that was first recognized in the belladonna plant. Atropine as we know it today was first purified by Mein in 1831. Its important effects on the cardiovascular system (the effects for which it is currently used) were recognized shortly thereafter.

Mechanism of Action

Atropine and related agents block the actions of acetylcholine (a neurotransmitter) at muscarinic receptors; hence the designation of these agents as muscarinic-cholinergic blockers or antimuscarinic agents. Since it is the release of acetylcholine from postganglionic autonomic nerves and its interaction with muscarinic receptors located on parasympathetic effector tissues (smooth muscle, heart tissue, exocrine glands) that mediate parasympathetic actions, agents (*e.g.,* atropine) that block this interaction function to inhibit parasympathetic responses (and hence are called *parasympatholytic* agents). The fact that not all body tissues are equally sensitive to the effects of atropine is clinically relevant. In general, the various glandular tissues (sweat, bronchial, and salivary glands) are most sensitive to the effects of atropine. Cardiac tissue is somewhat less sensitive, and the gastric parietal cells, along with several other tissues, are the least sensitive. Because the effects of atropine are both reversible and dose-dependent, the duration of its clinical effects may vary, and different doses may be required to produce desired clinical effects, depending on the degree of underlying parasympathetic stimulation.

Pharmacological Properties

Administration of atropine produces effects in the central nervous system, eyes, respiratory system, gastrointestinal system, genitourinary system, sweat glands, and, most important, from a prehospital perspective, in the cardiovascular system. Because the SA node, atria, and AV node receive significant parasympathetic innervation via the vagus nerve, these portions of the heart are particularly sensitive to the effects of atropine. Inhibition of vagal input to the SA node following the administration of atropine augments its rate of discharge and thereby increases heart rate. Similarly, decreased vagal input to the AV node increases conduction across this structure and facilitates transmission of impulses between the atria and ventricles. In sum, the important cardiovascular actions of atropine are to increase heart rate and to increase conduction across the AV node.

Pharmacokinetics

Atropine is widely distributed throughout the body, reaches significant concentrations within the central nervous system, and is cleared from the blood rapidly following administration. It has a half-life of approximately 2 hours and is excreted primarily through the kidneys.

Prehospital Indications

The major indications for use of atropine in the prehospital setting are sinus bradycardia associated with hemodynamic compromise; significant AV block; and asystole (use as one of several measures).

Side-Effects and Toxicity

Side-effects of atropine include drying of the mucous membranes and pupillary dilation. Toxic reactions include restlessness, altered mental status, irritability, and warm, dry, flushed skin.

Administration

In the prehospital setting, atropine is normally administered as a 0.5 mg rapid IV bolus that may be repeated up to a maximum dose of 2 mg.

increased rate of discharge from the sinus node. This latter effect can abolish many cases of sinus bradycardia. Administration normally involves an initial IV bolus of 0.5 mg, which may be repeated every 5 minutes if necessary, up to a maximum dose of 2 mg.

If clinically symptomatic sinus bradycardia persists despite treatment with atropine, consider further treatment using isoproterenol hydrochloride. Isoproterenol is a synthetic sympathomimetic agent that functions as a pure β-adrenergic agonist. Although its strong chronotropic properties (it increases heart rate) make it potentially useful in cases of bradycardia, it also has significant inotropic properties (it increases contractility) that may have adverse effects on the myocardium, especially in patients with underlying cardiac disease. For this reason, its use is restricted to those cases of clinically symptomatic sinus bradycardia that require correction but fail to respond to atropine. Administer an IV infusion at a rate of 2 to 10 ug/min and titrate to produce the desired clinical effect. Using isoproterenol is usually a temporary measure aimed at buying time until more definitive treatment, such as pacemaker therapy, can be carried out.

In our patient a beneficial clinical response follows the initial administration of atropine. Her improved mentation and normal blood pressure are accompanied by conversion of her cardiac rhythm from sinus bradycardia at a rate of 38 complexes per minute (Figure 16-1) to a normal sinus rhythm at a rate of 65 complexes per minute (Figure 16-2). Thus neither additional treatment with atropine nor use of isoproterenol are indicated. In summary, this elderly female patient experienced an acutely altered mental state and a syncopal episode. Her clinical picture included a slow sinus bradycardia and signs of hemodynamic instability, both of which responded well to treatment with atropine.

Field Diagnosis

- Hypotension and bradycardia
- Cardiac arrhythmia, sinus bradycardia with hemodynamic compromise

Hospital Diagnosis

- Sinus bradycardia corrected by atropine; etiology unknown

Patient Follow-Up

The patient was admitted for observation and further workup. A full 12 lead electrocardiogram revealed significant ST-segment elevations and T-wave inversions. Serial electrocardiograms and the results of cardiac enzyme measurement were consistent with the diagnosis of an extensive inferior wall myocardial infarction. The patient experienced an uneventful 10-day course in the hospital and was discharged with instructions for follow-up by her private physician.

Answers

1. A

    Josephine ME, Buxton AE, Marchlinski FE: The bradyarrhythmias. In Braunwald E, Isselbacher KJ, Petersdorf RG (eds): Harrison's Principles of Internal Medicine, 11th ed. New York, McGraw-Hill, 1987

    American Academy of Orthopaedic Surgeons: Emergency Care and Transportation of the Sick and Injured, 4th ed, pp 128–129. Menasha, WI, George Banta Co, 1987

2. D

    Huff J, Doernbach DP, White RD: ECG Workout: Exercises In Arrhythmia Interpretation, pp 36, 218 (strip 1.93). Philadelphia, JB Lippincott, 1985

    Chung EK: Principles of Cardiac Arrhythmias, 3rd ed, pp 58–63. Baltimore, Williams & Wilkins, 1983

    American Heart Association: Standards and guidelines for cardiopulmonary resuscitation (CPR) and emergency cardiac care (ECC). JAMA 255:2905, 1986

3. C

    Huff J, Doernbach DP, White RD: ECG Workout: Exercises In Arrhythmia Interpretation, pp 36, 218 (strip 1.93). Philadelphia, JB Lippincott, 1985

    Chung EK: Principles of Cardiac Arrhythmias, 3rd ed, pp 58–63. Baltimore, Williams & Wilkins, 1983

4. D

    Caroline NL: Emergency Care in the Streets, 3rd ed, pp 133–134, 286. Boston, Little, Brown & Co, 1987

    American Heart Association: Standards and guidelines for cardiopulmonary resuscitation (CPR) and emergency cardiac care (ECC). JAMA 255:2905 (see pages 2939, 2948–2949), 1986

5. A

    Huff J, Doernbach DP, White RD: ECG Workout: Exercises In Arrhythmia Interpretation, pp 24, 216 (strip 1.56). Philadelphia, JB Lippincott, 1985

6. D

    Caroline NL: Emergency Care in the Streets, 3rd ed, pp 133–134, 286. Boston, Little, Brown & Co, 1987

    American Heart Association: Standards and guidelines for cardiopulmonary resuscitation (CPR) and emergency cardiac care (ECC). JAMA 255:2905 (see pages 2939, 2948–2949), 1986

Selected Reading

American Heart Association: Standards and guidelines for cardiopulmonary resuscitation (CPR) and emergency cardiac care (ECC). JAMA 255:2905, 1986

17

Palpitations in a Middle-Aged Man

Your patient is an alert and oriented 48-year-old male who complains of nonradiating, substernal chest pain, which he describes as a "heavy pressure," and palpitations which began 4 hours ago and have persisted unabated. Past medical history is significant for diabetes mellitus treated with daily injections of insulin for the past 20 years. There is no significant family history and the patient denies any allergies. Physical examination is unremarkable except for a slightly pallid appearance and moderate diaphoresis. Vital signs are BP (right arm, sitting) 80/62, pulse 50 and irregular, and respiration 18 and regular.

1. Initial treatment should include
    1. Administering high-concentration oxygen
    2. Establishing an intravenous (IV) line
    3. Cardiac monitoring
    4. Administering morphine sulfate

    A. 1, 2, and 3 are correct
    B. 1 and 3 are correct
    C. 2 and 4 are correct
    D. Only 4 is correct
    E. All are correct

A1: Initial evaluation reveals a middle-aged man who presents with a combination of chest pain and palpitations. Physical assessment reveals two major areas of concern: a slow and irregular heart rate (50 beats per minute) and moderate hypotension. Although the etiology is unclear at this point, initial treatment should be directed towards hemodynamic stabilization. Administer supplemental oxygen to help correct any underlying hypoxia. Establish an IV line to serve as a medication and fluid route. Finally, institute cardiac monitoring as soon as possible to detect any cardiac arrhythmias. Although this patient has significant chest pain, the use of morphine sulfate at this point is inadvisable in view of the existing hypotension.

Following your initial treatment, cardiac monitoring shows the following cardiac rhythm (Figure 17–1):

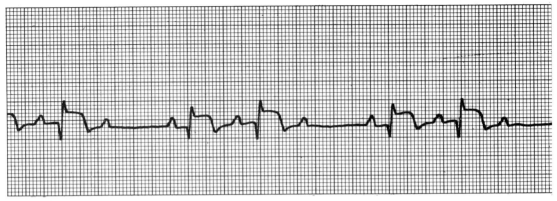

FIGURE 17-1

2. Abnormal findings on this tracing (Figure 17-1) include
   1. An irregular rhythm
   2. Nonconducted atrial impulses
   3. An elevated ST segment
   4. Abnormally prolonged QRS complexes

   A. 1, 2, and 3 are correct
   B. 1 and 3 are correct
   C. 2 and 4 are correct
   D. Only 4 is correct
   E. All are correct

3. This rhythm (Figure 17-1) is best classified as
   A. Third degree AV block
   B. Atrial fibrillation
   C. Second degree AV block, Mobitz type I
   D. Normal sinus rhythm with nonconducted premature atrial contractions
   E. Second degree AV block, Mobitz type II

A2 and 3: Examination of this tracing reveals an irregular rhythm with an atrial rate of 83, a ventricular rate of 50, and significant elevation of the ST segment. Careful inspection of the tracing shows that while each QRS complex is preceded by a P wave, not every P wave is followed by a QRS complex. This disparity between the atrial P waves and the ventricular QRS complexes suggests some form of heart block. Further analysis shows a cyclic pattern in which the PR interval increases in length (from 0.20 sec to 0.24 sec) and is followed by a nonconducted P wave. This pattern defines the presence of a *Mobitz type I (Wenckebach) AV block*, a form of second degree AV block. This arrhythmia may be seen in several conditions (see "Etiology of Mobitz type I, Second Degree AV Block"), but its most important clinical correlation is with acute myocardial infarction (AMI). More specifically, Mobitz type I AV block is often associated with acute diaphragmatic (inferior) wall myocardial infarction. This association is explained by the fact

Etiology of Mobitz type I, Second Degree AV Block

- Increased vagal stimulation
- Digitalis intoxication
- Quinidine intoxication
- Rheumatic heart disease
- Acute myocardial infarction (commonly inferior wall infarcts)

that in the majority of persons the right coronary artery provides blood to both the AV junction and the inferior wall of the myocardium; therefore, occlusion of this artery can produce the combination of inferior wall myocardial infarction and Mobitz type I AV block.

4. Treatment of your patient's initial cardiac rhythm (Figure 17-1) calls for
   A. Bretylium tosylate, 300 mg, IV bolus
   B. Calcium chloride, 5 ml of a 10% solution, IV bolus
   C. Atropine sulfate, 0.5 mg, IV bolus
   D. Sodium bicarbonate, 88 mEq, IV bolus

A4: Initial treatment of your patient's cardiac arrhythmias is indicated in view of the associated clinical symptoms (chest pain, hypotension, and extremely slow ventricular rate). The initial treatment of choice in the prehospital setting is atropine sulfate, a parasympatholytic agent that acts both to promote atrioventricular conduction and to increase the rate of sinus node discharge. In cases of sinus bradycardia or AV block associated with hemodynamic compromise, the recommended initial dose of atropine sulfate is 0.5 mg IV.

Following treatment your patient's cardiac rhythm remains unchanged (Figure 17-1) and his chest pain and hypotension continue. Vital signs are BP 78/64, pulse 52 and irregular, and respiration 14 and regular.

5. Appropriate treatment at this point might include
   A. Defibrillation at 360 J
   B. Atropine sulfate, 0.5 mg, IV bolus
   C. Bretylium tosylate, 300 mg, IV bolus
   D. Calcium chloride, 5 ml of a 10% solution, IV bolus
   E. Morphine sulfate, 5 mg, slow IV push

A5: At this point your patient has received only a single 0.5 mg IV bolus of atropine sulfate. Because full vagal blockade may not result until 2 mg of atropine have been administered, a repeat bolus of atropine sulfate, 0.5 mg IV, is indicated. Current recommendations include administering atropine sulfate as a 0.5 mg bolus every 5 minutes until either clinical improvement results or a total dose of 2 mg has been administered.

Following the second bolus of atropine sulfate, your patient reports that his chest pain, although still present, has diminished somewhat in intensity. Vital signs are BP (right arm, sitting) 98/78, pulse 72 and irregular, and respiration 14 and regular. Cardiac monitoring shows the following (Figure 17-2):

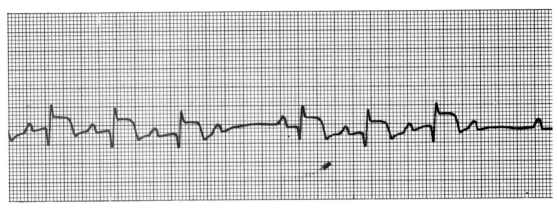

FIGURE 17-2

6. This tracing (Figure 17-2) demonstrates a(n)
   1. Atrial rate of approximately 90 beats per minute
   2. QRS duration of approximately .08 seconds
   3. Variation in the PR interval
   4. Ventricular rate of approximately 70 beats per minute

   A. 1, 2, and 3 are correct
   B. 1 and 3 are correct
   C. 2 and 4 are correct
   D. Only 4 is correct
   E. All are correct

7. Correct interpretation of this rhythm (Figure 17-2) is
   A. Normal sinus rhythm with nonconducted premature atrial contractions
   B. Second degree AV block, Mobitz type I
   C. Normal sinus rhythm with multiple premature ventricular contractions
   D. Third degree AV block
   E. Atrial fibrillation with rapid ventricular response

A6 and 7: Your patient's EKG continues to show a Mobitz type I AV block. However, the ventricular rate has now increased to approximately 70 beats per minute, probably as a result of increased AV conduction secondary to the administration of atropine.

8. Treatment at this point should include
   A. Isoproterenol hydrochloride, 2 to10 ug/min, IV infusion
   B. Calcium chloride, 5 ml of a 10% solution, IV bolus
   C. Bretylium tosylate, 300 mg, IV bolus

D. Sodium bicarbonate, 44 mEq, IV bolus
E. None of the above

A8: No further medications are required at this point since your patient appears hemodynamically stable and clinically improved. In view of the possibility of myocardial infarction, however, continuous cardiac monitoring, frequent evaluation of vital signs, and continued oxygen administration are in order, along with rapid transport to a medical facility.

Field Diagnosis

- Mobitz type I second degree AV block
- Symptomatic hypotension

Hospital Diagnosis

- Acute inferior wall myocardial infarction
- Mobitz type I second degree AV block

Patient Follow-Up

The patient was admitted to the cardiac intensive care unit for observation and further evaluation. Electrocardiograms and serial cardiac enzyme measurements confirmed the suspicion of an inferior wall myocardial infarction. Although the patient suffered persistent cardiac arrhythmias associated with hemodynamic instability for several days, his condition finally stabilized and he was discharged after 10 days in the hospital.

Answers

1. A

    American Heart Association: Standards and guidelines for cardiopulmonary resuscitation (CPR) and emergency cardiac care (ECC). JAMA 255:2905 (see pp 2944–2945, 2948–2949), 1986

    Caroline NL: Emergency Care in the Streets, 3rd ed, pp 264–265. Boston, Little, Brown & Co, 1987

2. A

    Huff J, Doernbach DP, White RD: ECG Workout: Exercises in Arrhythmia Interpretation, pp 104, 233 (strip 3.74). Philadelphia, JB Lippincott, 1985

3. C

    Huff J, Doernbach DP, White RD: ECG Workout: Exercises in Arrhythmia Interpretation, pp 104, 233 (strip 3.74). Philadelphia, JB Lippincott, 1985

    Caroline NL: Emergency Care in the Streets, 3rd ed, pp 294–295. Boston, Little, Brown & Co, 1987

    Josephson ME, Buxton AE, Marchlinksi FE: The bradyarrhythmias. In Braunwald E, Isselbacher KJ, Petersdorf RG (eds): Harrison's Principles of Internal Medicine, 11th ed, p 921. New York, McGraw-Hill, 1987

4. C

    Caroline NL: Emergency Care in the Streets, 3rd ed, pp 133–134, 286, 294–295. Boston, Little, Brown & Co, 1987

    American Heart Association: Standards and guidelines for cardiopulmonary resuscitation (CPR) and emergency cardiac care (ECC). JAMA 255:2905 (see pages 2944, 2948–2949), 1986

5. B

Caroline NL: Emergency Care in the Streets, 3rd ed, pp 133–134, 286, 294–295. Boston, Little, Brown & Co, 1987

American Heart Association: Standards and guidelines for cardiopulmonary resuscitation (CPR) and emergency cardiac care (ECC). JAMA 255:2905 (see pages 2944, 2948–2949), 1986

6. E

Huff J, Doernbach DP, White RD: ECG Workout: Exercises in Arrhythmia Interpretation, pp 100, 232 (strip 3.63). Philadelphia, JB Lippincott, 1985

7. B

Huff J, Doernbach DP, White RD: ECG Workout: Exercises in Arrhythmia Interpretation, pp 100, 232 (strip 3.63). Philadelphia, JB Lippincott, 1985

8. E

American Heart Association: Standards and guidelines for cardiopulmonary resuscitation (CPR) and emergency cardiac care (ECC). JAMA 255:2905 (see page 2944), 1986

Caroline NL: Emergency Care in the Streets, 3rd ed, p 286. Boston, Little, Brown & Co, 1987

Selected Reading

American Heart Association: Standards and guidelines for cardiopulmonary resuscitation (CPR) and emergency cardiac care (ECC). JAMA 255:2905, 1986

18

Acute Chest Pain Followed by Cardiopulmonary Arrest

You are called to evaluate the condition of an elderly woman who called EMS complaining of chest pain. Upon arrival at the scene, you encounter a 68-year-old woman who is sitting upright and who appears severely diaphoretic and in moderate distress. Upon questioning, she reports severe retrosternal chest pain that radiates to the left and right arms and that began 1 hour ago. She describes the pain as a "deep pressurelike" feeling that has been constant since its onset. She has had no history of similar episodes and could not obtain relief by taking either antacids or aspirin. She is extremely nauseous and vomited twice shortly after the pain began.

The patient has no history of recent trauma, fever, chronic obstructive pulmonary disease, heart disease, or diabetes. She does admit to a long history of hypertension for which she takes hydrochlorothiazide, 25 mg po bid, and clonidine, 0.3 mg po bid. She denies any allergies, does not smoke, and admits to being a "social" drinker. Family history is remarkable only for the premature death of her sister at age 45 from what the patient describes only as "heart problems."

Physical examination reveals an alert and oriented, severely diaphoretic, and extremely agitated woman. Vital signs are BP (right arm, sitting) 98/64, pulse 50 weak and irregular, and respiration 24 regular and full. The head and neck are without signs of trauma, the trachea is midline, and no bruits are noted. Sclera are nonicteric, although the conjunctiva are pallid. The thorax shows symmetrical respiratory excursion. Breath sounds are clear bilaterally without rales, rhonchi, or wheezes. Heart sounds are S_1S_2 and clear, with an irregular rhythm at a rate of 46 beats per minute. There is no evidence of jugular venous distension (JVD) or hepatojugular reflux (HJR).

The abdomen is soft and nontender without pain, tenderness, or guarding. Bowel sounds are auscultated in all quadrants. The extremities are cool and pallid with poor capillary refill in the nail beds. Distal pulses are symmetrical in all extremities. No clubbing, cyanosis, or edema are noted. Neurologically, the patient is alert and oriented to time, place, and self. Pupils are round, equal, and reactive to light. Spontaneous movements and good muscle strength are present in all extremities. Repeat vital signs reveal BP (right arm, supine) 82/70, and pulse 48 weak and irregular. No orthostatic changes are present.

1. Initial treatment should include all the following except
    A. Establishing an intravenous (IV) line
    B. Administering supplemental oxygen
    C. Cardiac monitoring
    D. Applying venous constricting bands (VCBs)

A1: This patient presents with a clinical history that strongly suggests acute myocardial infarction (AMI). Initial treatment should be oriented toward better defining the etiology of the patient's problems and supporting vital body functions. Establishing an IV line is essential in order to facilitate both medication and fluid administration. In cases of suspected AMI, administer supplemental oxygen via face mask or nasal cannula at 4 to 6 l/min to ensure adequate arterial oxygen tension and hemoglobin saturation. The initial use of morphine sulfate is not called for here, in view of your patient's significant hypotensive state (BP 82/70). Cardiac monitoring is essential to better define the nature of your patient's condition.

Your patient's initial cardiac rhythm reveals the following (Figure 18-1):

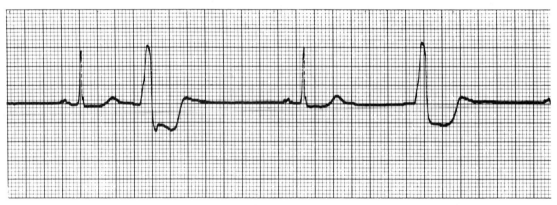

FIGURE 18-1

2. The initial cardiac rhythm (Figure 18-1) shows
    A. Complete third degree AV block
    B. Sinus bradycardia with premature ventricular beats
    C. Agonal idioventricular rhythm
    D. Sinus arrhythmia with premature atrial contractions

A2: Inspection of the initial EKG tracing shows an irregular rhythm with a rate of approximately 50 beats per minute. The first, third, and fifth complexes appear to be of sinus origin, with each possessing a P wave, normal PR interval, QRS complex of normal duration (.06 sec) and morphology, and normally placed T waves. In contrast, the second and fourth complexes show several abnormal features: they occur prematurely in the cycle, are wide and bizarre in shape, have oppositely directed T waves, and are not preceded by distinct P waves. These characteristics suggest a ventricular origin for these complexes, and a full interpretation of this EKG would be underlying sinus bradycardia with associated premature ventricular beats.

3. Correct treatment at this point calls for administering
   A. Lidocaine, 100 mg bolus with a 2 mg/min drip
   B. Bretylium tosylate, 300 mg, IV bolus
   C. Atropine sulfate, 0.5 mg, IV bolus
   D. Calcium chloride, 2 ml of a 10% solution

A3: Treatment at this stage is aimed at improving your patient's hemodynamic status. In view of the clinically significant bradycardia, the drug of choice is atropine sulfate, 0.5 mg, IV bolus. Although premature ventricular contractions are also present, the use of lidocaine is not initially called for to treat hemodynamically significant bradycardia with coexisting premature ventricular beats. Rather, a parasympatholytic agent such as atropine may help to increase sinus node discharge and improve cardiac output.

Shortly after the administration of atropine, your patient suddenly becomes unconscious. Rapid assessment reveals absence of spontaneous respiration and no palpable pulse. The cardiac monitor shows the following (Figure 18-2):

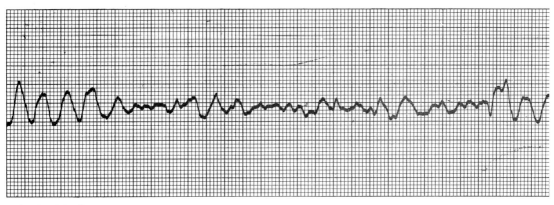

FIGURE 18-2

4. The patient's EKG at this point (Figure 18-2) demonstrates
   A. Ventricular tachycardia
   B. Atrial fibrillation
   C. Ventricular fibrillation
   D. Complete third degree AV block

A4: This totally chaotic rhythm without any discernable complexes indicates ventricular fibrillation. Although lead placement should always be checked to rule out the possibility of artifact or a detached electrode, the patient's unresponsiveness along with this EKG pattern leaves little question that the existing arrhythmia is ventricular fibrillation.

5. Immediate treatment calls for
   A. Precordial thump and immediate defibrillation
   B. Immediate administration of lidocaine, 100 mg IV bolus, followed by cardiopulmonary resuscitation (CPR)
   C. Immediate intubation followed by defibrillation
   D. Application of military antishock trousers (MAST) and CPR

A5: Because ventricular fibrillation is universally fatal unless rapidly corrected, immediate treatment is in order. In cases of witnessed and confirmed cardiopulmonary arrest, current recommendations call for administering an initial precordial thump, CPR until a defibrillator is available, and then immediate defibrillation (see "Precordial Thump Technique" and "Defibrillation Technique").

Precordial Thump Technique

Indications

- Monitored ventricular fibrillation
- Monitored pulseless ventricular tachycardia
- Asystole
- Witnessed cardiac arrest with no available defibrillator

Technique

- Hold closed fist 8-12 inches over patient's chest
- Strike midportion of the sternum with the hypothenar eminence
- Deliver as a single, sharp, rapid blow

Proposed Mechanism of Action

- Produces a "mechanical defibrillation" by effecting a low energy (2-5 Joule) depolarization

Potential Complications

- Fractures of the sternum and ribs
- Conversion to a more malignant rhythm (*i.e.*, ventricular tachycardia with a pulse, to ventricular fibrillation)

Defibrillation Technique

- Apply conductive gel to paddles
- Turn synchronize mode to "off" position
- Turn defibrillator power "on"
- Set desired energy level and charge machine
- Position paddles correctly over chest
- ENSURE ALL PERSONNEL ARE CLEAR, MAKING SURE THEY ARE NOT IN DIRECT OR INDIRECT CONTACT WITH THE PATIENT
- Recheck cardiac rhythm on monitor
- Depress both discharge buttons simultaneously to deliver countershock

Following your initial attempt at defibrillation your patient is still pulseless and the cardiac monitor shows the following (Figure 18–3):

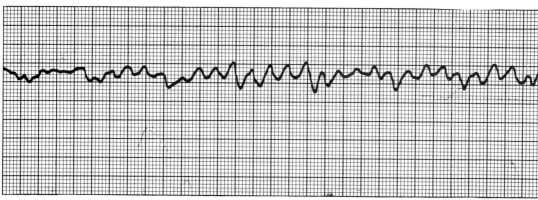

FIGURE 18–3

6. The next step should be
    A. Immediate delivery of a precordial thump
    B. Administration of bretylium tosylate, 500 mg, IV bolus
    C. Immediate defibrillation at 200 to 300 Joules
    D. Administration of lidocaine, 100 mg, IV bolus

A6: Your patient remains unresponsive and the EKG shows ventricular fibrillation (Figure 18–3). Although your initial attempt at defibrillation was unsuccessful, a second attempt is called for. Current work has shown that rapid defibrillation is the single most important factor in effecting survival in cases of out-of-hospital ventricular fibrillation. For this reason, current recommendations call for the delivery of three sequential and consecutive countershocks in rapid sequence, before other measures are undertaken. The initial defibrillation should deliver 200 Joules, the second attempt 200 to 300 Joules, and the third attempt 360 Joules.

Following the second and then the third attempt at defibrillation, the patient remains unresponsive without spontaneous respiration or a palpable pulse, and with a cardiac rhythm still showing ventricular fibrillation.

7. At this point appropriate steps include all the following except
    A. CPR
    B. Establishment of IV access
    C. Administration of epinephrine 1:10,000, 0.5 mg to 1 mg via intracardiac injection
    D. Endotracheal intubation

A7: In the face of continued ventricular fibrillation and three unsuccessful preliminary attempts at defibrillation, institute (or continue) CPR while IV access and endotracheal intubation are attempted. As soon as IV access has been gained the medication of choice is epinephrine, 1:10,000, 0.5 mg to 1 mg, IV bolus. If no IV line can be accessed, then administer epinephrine by an endotracheal tube in a dose of 1 mg (10 ml of a 1:10,000 solution). The administration of epinephrine as an intracardiac injection has fallen out of use, due to the numerous complications with which it is associated (e.g., pneumothorax, cardiac tamponade, laceration of the coronary arteries); use only if no other access routes exist.

Cardiopulmonary resuscitation is continued but the patient remains unresponsive, without either spontaneous respiration or a spontaneous pulse. The cardiac monitor now shows the following (Figure 18-4):

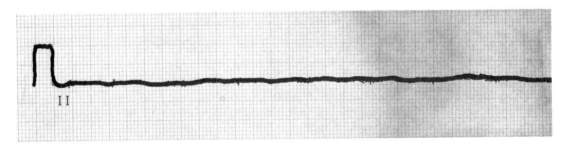

FIGURE 18-4

8. Correct steps at this point include all the following except
   A. Check that all monitor leads are intact
   B. Switch to another lead to confirm rhythm
   C. Administer atropine sulfate, 1 mg IV push
   D. Administer lidocaine, 100 mg, IV push

A8: The patient's cardiac rhythm shows a pattern of asystole (Figure 18-4). Although asystole is easy to recognize, two situations that may masquerade as asystole must always be considered. First, ensure that there are no loose or displaced electrodes; these can create a false picture of asystole on the cardiac monitor. Second, fine ventricular fibrillation may resemble asystole when one is looking at a single EKG lead (as is common practice during a code situation). Always switch to a second lead to confirm that asystole and not fine ventricular fibrillation is occurring. Once asystole has been confirmed, the treatment of choice is epinephrine, 1:10,000, 0.5 to 1 mg IV bolus, followed by atropine, 1 mg IV bolus.

Following the above measures your patient continues to demonstrate asystole. Medical control is contacted and 45 minutes into the code a joint decision is made to halt further resuscitative efforts.

Answers

1. **D**
   Caroline NL: Emergency Care in the Streets, 3rd ed, pp 264–269. Boston, Little, Brown & Co, 1987
   Grauer K, Cavallaro D: ACLS: Certification Preparation and a Comprehensive Review, 2nd ed, pp 260–262. St Louis, CV Mosby, 1987
   American Heart Association: Standards and guidelines for cardiopulmonary resuscitation (CPR) and emergency cardiac care (ECC). JAMA 255:2905 (see page 2944), 1986

2. **B**
   Huff J, Doernbach DP, White RD: ECG Workout: Exercises in Arrhythmia Interpretation, pp 128, 238 (strip 4.33). Philadelphia, JB Lippincott, 1985
   Caroline NL: Emergency Care in the Streets, 3rd ed, pp 286, 297. Boston, Little, Brown & Co, 1987

3. **C**
   American Heart Association: Standards and guidelines for cardiopulmonary resuscitation (CPR) and emergency cardiac care (ECC). JAMA 255:2905 (see pages 2945, 2948–2949), 1986
   Caroline NL: Emergency Care in the Streets, 3rd ed, p 286. Boston, Little, Brown & Co, 1987

4. **C**
   Huff J, Doernbach DP, White RD: ECG Workout: Exercises in Arrhythmia Interpretation, pp 119, 236 (strip 4.5). Philadelphia, JB Lippincott, 1985
   Caroline NL: Emergency Care in the Streets, 3rd ed, p 300. Boston, Little, Brown & Co, 1987

5. **A**
   American Heart Association: Standards and guidelines for cardiopulmonary resuscitation (CPR) and emergency cardiac care (ECC). JAMA 255:2905 (see pages 2942, 2945–2946), 1986
   Caroline NL: Emergency Care in the Streets, 3rd ed, p 300. Boston, Little, Brown & Co, 1987

6. **C**
   American Heart Association: Standards and guidelines for cardiopulmonary resuscitation (CPR) and emergency cardiac care (ECC). JAMA 255:2905 (see pages 2942, 2945–2946), 1986
   Caroline NL: Emergency Care in the Streets, 3rd ed, pp 326–329. Boston, Little, Brown & Co, 1987

7. **C**
   American Heart Association: Standards and guidelines for cardiopulmonary resuscitation (CPR) and emergency cardiac care (ECC). JAMA 255:2905 (see page 2940), 1986

8. **D**
   American Heart Association: Standards and guidelines for cardiopulmonary resuscitation (CPR) and emergency cardiac care (ECC). JAMA 255:2905 (see page 2947), 1986
   Caroline NL: Emergency Care in the Streets, 3rd ed, p 331. Boston, Little, Brown & Co, 1987

Selected Reading

American Heart Association: Standards and guidelines for cardiopulmonary resuscitation (CPR) and emergency cardiac care (ECC). JAMA 255:2905, 1986

19

Cardiac Arrest with Multiple Malignant Arrhythmias

You are called to report to the scene of a fire following a report of a fireman in cardiac arrest. Upon arrival, you find a somewhat obese, middle-aged man sprawled out on the ground, unconscious and unresponsive. Cardiopulmonary resuscitation (CPR) is being performed and an intravenous (IV) line is in place. The scene commander informs you that the patient collapsed approximately 10 minutes ago, and that CPR was immediately instituted. A quick assessment reveals no spontaneous pulse, respiration, or blood pressure. Cardiopulmonary resuscitation is being performed adequately. After initiating cardiac monitoring you see the following (Figure 19–1):

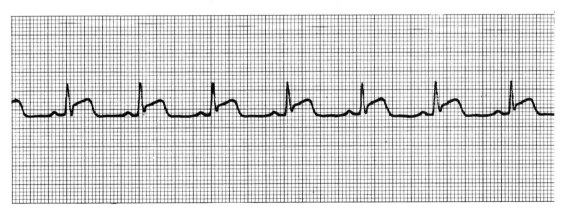

FIGURE 19–1

1. This tracing most accurately reflects
    A. Sinus tachycardia
    B. Second degree AV block
    C. Electromechanical dissociation
    D. Ventricular fibrillation

A1: In the above tracing we see a clear-cut sinus rhythm, although there is no

181

evidence of any mechanical cardiac activity (no pulse or blood pressure). The finding of organized electrical activity on the EKG in the absence of effective mechanical activity is known as electromechanical dissociation (EMD).

2. Treatment of your patient at this point should include
   A. Immediate defibrillation
   B. Lidocaine, 100 mg, IV bolus
   C. Calcium chloride, 2 ml of a 10% solution
   D. Epinephrine, 1:10,000, 0.5 to 1 mg, IV bolus

A2: Treatment of EMD calls for initiating CPR, establishing IV access (and intubating, if feasible), and administering epinephrine, 1:10,000, 0.5 mg to 1 mg, as an IV bolus. Repeat at 5-minute intervals as required.

3. Potentially correctable causes of EMD include which of the following?
   1. Hypoxemia
   2. Pericardial tamponade
   3. Tension pneumothorax
   4. Pulmonary embolism

   A. 1, 2, and 3 are correct
   B. 1 and 3 are correct
   C. 2 and 4 are correct
   D. Only 4 is correct
   E. All are correct

A3: All of the above conditions may produce EMD. Because EMD carries with it a poor prognosis, make every attempt to detect and correct any potentially treatable cause (see "Potentially Correctable Causes of EMD").

Potentially Correctable Causes of EMD

- Pulmonary embolism
- Hypoxemia
- Tension pneumothorax
- Pericardial tamponade
- Hypovolemia
- Metabolic derangements

Ten minutes into the arrest your patient remains without a palpable pulse or spontaneous respiration, but develops the rhythm shown below (Figure 19-2):

4. This rhythm is best classified as
   A. Ventricular fibrillation
   B. Asystole
   C. Sinus arrhythmia
   D. Ventricular tachycardia

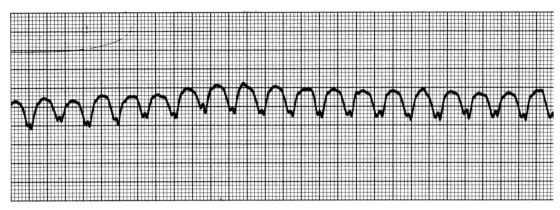

FIGURE 19-2

A4: This tracing (Figure 19-2) shows a regular rhythm at a rate of approximately 188 beats per minute. Discrete P waves are not seen and the QRS complexes are prolonged to 0.16 seconds. Proper interpretation of this tracing is ventricular tachycardia.

5. Treatment at this point should include
   A. Defibrillation
   B. Administration of atropine sulfate, 0.5 mg, IV bolus
   C. Administration of bretylium tosylate, 500 mg, IV push
   D. Administration of epinephrine, 1:10,000, 0.5 to 1 mg, IV bolus

A5: Treatment of pulseless ventricular tachycardia is identical to treatment of ventricular fibrillation. Immediate defibrillation starting with 200 Joules is indicated. If this is unsuccessful, attempt a second and third defibrillation with progressively increasing energy levels (200 to 300 Joules for the second attempt and 360 Joules for the third attempt).

Following your initial defibrillation attempt, the patient regains a spontaneous pulse and blood pressure and displays the following cardiac rhythm (Figure 19-3):

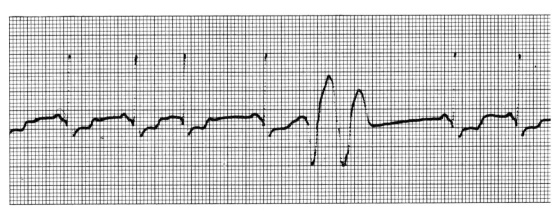

FIGURE 19-3

Vital signs at this point are BP 100/76, pulse 80 weak and irregular, and respiration 12 and regular.

6. Treatment at this point should include
   A. Atropine sulfate, 0.5 mg, IV push
   B. Lidocaine, 100 mg, IV bolus with a 2 mg/min drip
   C. Epinephrine, 1:10,000, 0.5 to 1 mg, IV push
   D. Calcium chloride, 2 ml of a 10% solution

A6: Careful examination of the patient's cardiac rhythm shows an underlying sinus rhythm with a single premature atrial beat (fourth complex) and paired premature ventricular beats. Associated with this are an adequate blood pressure and spontaneous respiration. Treatment at this point should include administering a 1 mg/kg lidocaine bolus followed by a lidocaine drip at 2 mg/min.

Field Diagnosis

- Cardiopulmonary arrest

Hospital Diagnosis

- Status postcardiopulmonary arrest
- Acute anterior wall myocardial infarction

Patient Follow-Up

When your patient was evaluated in the emergency room, a 12 lead EKG demonstrated evidence of an acute anterior wall myocardial infarction. Cardiac enzymes were drawn and measured, appropriate lab work and tests were carried out, and the patient was immediately transferred to the cardiac care unit. Aggressive treatment with antiarrhythmic agents was required during the first 24 hours to manage a variety of malignant cardiac arrhythmias. On the second day in the hospital the patient coded twice; he was successfully resuscitated both times. Following a complicated two-week hospital stay, your patient was discharged and scheduled for follow-up care with his private medical doctor.

Answers

1. C

Caroline NL: Emergency Care in the Streets, 3rd ed, pp 315, 331. Boston, Little, Brown & Co, 1987

Huff J, Doernbach DP, White RD: ECG Workout: Exercises in Arrhythmia Interpretation, pp 31, 217 (strip 1.77). Philadelphia, JB Lippincott, 1985

American Heart Association: Standards and guidelines for cardiopulmonary resuscitation (CPR) and emergency cardiac care (ECC). JAMA 255:2905 (see page 2948), 1986

2. D

Caroline NL: Emergency Care in the Streets, 3rd ed, pp 331. Boston, Little, Brown & Co, 1987

American Heart Association: Standards and guidelines for cardiopulmonary resuscitation (CPR) and emergency cardiac care (ECC). JAMA 255:2905 (see pages 2947-2948), 1986

Grauer K, Cavallaro D: ACLS: Certification Preparation and a Comprehensive Review, 2nd ed, pp 14-15. St Louis, CV Mosby, 1987

3. E

Caroline NL: Emergency Care in the Streets, 3rd ed, p 331. Boston, Little, Brown & Co, 1987

American Heart Association: Standards and guidelines for cardiopulmonary resuscitation (CPR) and emergency cardiac care (ECC). JAMA 255:2905 (see pages 2947-2948), 1986

Grauer K, Cavallaro D: ACLS: Certification Preparation and a Comprehensive Review, 2nd ed, pp 14-15. St Louis, CV Mosby, 1987

4. D

Huff J, Doernbach DP, White RD: ECG Workout: Exercises in Arrhythmia Interpretation, pp 126, 238 (strip 4.25). Philadelphia, JB Lippincott, 1985

5. A

Grauer K, Cavallaro D: ACLS: Certification Preparation and a Comprehensive Review, 2nd ed, pp 9-10. St Louis, CV Mosby, 1987

American Heart Association: Standards and guidelines for cardiopulmonary resuscitation (CPR) and emergency cardiac care (ECC). JAMA 255:2905 (see pp 2946-2947), 1986

6. B

American Heart Association: Standards and guidelines for cardiopulmonary resuscitation (CPR) and emergency cardiac care (ECC). JAMA 255:2905 (see p 2949), 1986

Caroline NL: Emergency Care in the Streets, 3rd ed, p 297-298. Boston, Little, Brown & Co, 1987

Grauer K, Cavallaro D: ACLS: Certification Preparation and a Comprehensive Review, 2nd ed, pp 275-287. St Louis, CV Mosby, 1987

Selected Reading

American Heart Association: Standards and guidelines for cardiopulmonary resuscitation (CPR) and emergency cardiac care (ECC). JAMA 255:2905, 1986

20

Dizziness in an Elderly Man

Your patient is a 75-year-old man who lives alone and has called EMS complaining of dizziness. You find him supine on the kitchen floor, responsive to verbal stimuli, but confused and unable to provide you with a clear medical history. There are no signs of trauma, and physical examination is unremarkable except for cyanosis and delayed capillary refill in the fingernail beds. Vital signs are BP (left arm, supine) 80/56, pulse 32 weak and regular, and respiration 12 and regular. You begin cardiac monitoring and see the following rhythm (Figure 20–1):

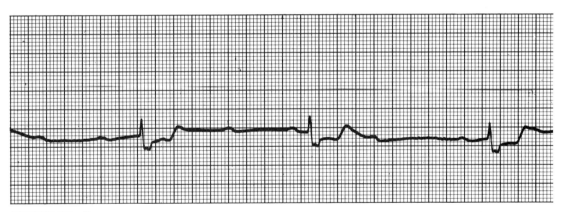

FIGURE 20–1

1. The patient's initial cardiac rhythm (Figure 20–1) is best classified as
   A. Sinus bradycardia
   B. Second degree AV block, Mobitz type I
   C. Third degree AV block
   D. Second degree AV block, Mobitz type II
   E. Sinus bradycardia with premature ventricular contractions

2. Initial patient management is best accomplished by
   1. Administration of high-concentration oxygen
   2. Endotracheal intubation

187

3. Establishment of an intravenous line
4. Inflation of MAST

A. 1, 2, and 3 are correct
B. 1 and 3 are correct
C. 2 and 4 are correct
D. Only 4 is correct
E. All are correct

3. Medical management of the patient's cardiac rhythm (Figure 20–1) calls for
   A. Lidocaine, 75 to 100 mg, IV bolus, followed by a 2 to 4 mg/min infusion
   B. Bretylium tosylate, 10 mg, IV bolus, followed by a 2 mg/min infusion
   C. Atropine sulfate, 0.5 to 1 mg, IV bolus
   D. Calcium chloride, 5 ml of a 10% solution, IV bolus
   E. Morphine sulfate, 5 mg, slow IV push

The patient remains confused and complains of weakness and dizziness. Repeat vital signs at this point are BP (left arm, supine) 82/60, pulse 34 weak and regular, and respiration 10 and regular. His cardiac rhythm is unchanged (Figure 20–1).

4. At this point appropriate medical treatment calls for
   A. Atropine sulfate, 0.5 to 1 mg, IV bolus
   B. Lidocaine, 75 mg, IV bolus
   C. Morphine sulfate, 2 mg, slow IV push
   D. Magnesium sulfate, 4 g, slow IV push
   E. None of the above

The patient continues to exhibit serious confusion and a blood pressure of 76/54. Cardiac monitoring shows the following (Figure 20–2):

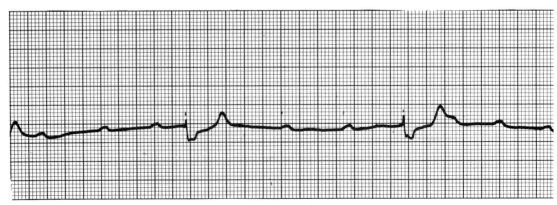

FIGURE 20–2

5. You reestablish contact with medical control and they request your interpretation of the cardiac rhythm (Figure 20-2). Your best response would be
   A. Atrial fibrillation with slow ventricular response
   B. Second degree AV block, Mobitz type I
   C. Sinus bradycardia with nonconducted premature atrial contractions
   D. Second degree AV block, Mobitz type II
   E. Third degree AV block

6. After discussion with medical control a decision is made to administer a second medication, most probably
   A. Lidocaine, 75 to 100 mg IV bolus, followed by a 2 to 4 mg/min infusion
   B. Isoproterenol, 2 to 10 ug/min, IV infusion
   C. Calcium chloride, 5 ml of a 10% solution, IV bolus
   D. Atropine, 5 mg, IV slow push
   E. Verapamil, 10 mg, IV push

The patient's cardiac rhythm remains unchanged (Figure 20-2) and he continues to be disoriented and hypotensive. Transport to a nearby hospital is undertaken and cardiac monitoring continues.

7. Definitive in-hospital treatment of the patient's cardiac arrhythmia will most likely involve
   A. Defibrillation at 360 J
   B. An artificial cardiac pacemaker
   C. Synchronized cardioversion at 25 J
   D. Immediate cardiac surgery

Discussion

An elderly man presents with an altered mental state, cyanosis, and serious hypotension. Although these findings may reflect a variety of conditions, the extremely slow pulse rate (32 beats per minute) implies a cardiac arrhythmia as either a primary or secondary phenomenon in the etiology of the patient's condition.

The initial cardiac tracing (Figure 20-1) reveals a third degree AV heart block. The atrial rate is roughly 70 beats per minute, while the ventricular rate is only 30 beats per minute. There is no constant PR interval and no apparent relationship between the atrial P waves and the ventricular QRS complexes. In *third degree AV block,* also known as complete heart block, the AV tissue fails to transmit atrial impulses to the ventricles. In most cases, a back-up pacemaker below the site of the block will substitute to stimulate ventricular activity. The result is that both an atrial and ventricular rhythm will usually be present, but will be independent of each other, each being controlled by a separate pacemaker. Complete AV dissociation is said to exist since there is no relationship between the observed atrial and ventricular activity.

The atrial rhythm may vary from normal depolarization via the SA node to any of several ectopic tachycardias, including atrial fibrillation, atrial flutter, and atrial tachycardia. In this particular tracing, the P waves are of normal morphology and occur at a rate of approximately 70 waves per minute. These findings suggest that normal discharge from the SA node is responsible for the observed atrial rhythm.

The type of ventricular rhythm seen in third degree AV block depends on which portion of the conduction system substitutes to pace the ventricles. If the back-up pacemaker lies above the bifurcation of the bundle of His, the resulting ventricular complexes are usually of normal duration and morphology, with a rate characteristically between 40 and 60 beats per minute. This type of rhythm is called an *AV junctional escape rhythm*. If, on the other hand, the pacemaker lies below the bifurcation of the bundle of His, then the QRS complexes commonly have a wide and bizarre shape and a slower rate, usually less than 40 beats per minute. This is called a *ventricular escape rhythm* or *idioventricular rhythm*.

In this tracing (Figure 20-1) the QRS complexes show a prolonged duration between 0.12 and 0.14 seconds and a slow rate of approximately 30 complexes per minute, findings that suggest a ventricular escape rhythm. Although a full cardiogram must be viewed to rule out the possibility of an AV junctional escape rhythm with aberrant conduction, based on the available information a full description of the patient's initial cardiac arrhythmia (Figure 20-1) is *third degree AV block with an atrial rhythm of sinus origin and a ventricular escape rhythm (idioventricular rhythm) at 32 complexes per minute*.

The hemodynamic effects of this arrhythmia largely depend on the ventricular rate and the pumping ability of the heart muscle. A slow ventricular rate, as in this patient, coupled with a weakened myocardium, can lead to a serious decrease in cardiac output. This condition is reflected in the patient's altered mental state, hypotension, and cyanosis.

Initial treatment of the patient calls for administering high-concentration oxygen to maintain adequate oxygenation, and immediately establishing an intravenous (IV) line to serve as a fluid and medication route. For the patient with third degree AV block, the decision to administer medications to correct the arrhythmia depends on two key factors: the ventricular rate and the clinical status of the patient. When there is a ventricular rate of less than 60 beats per minute and symptoms of hemodynamic compromise (*i.e.*, hypotension), as in the present case, medical treatment is called for (Table 20-1).

The initial medication of choice is atropine sulfate administered as a 0.5-1 mg IV bolus. Reevaluate the cardiac rhythm and if no change has taken place, administer a repeat bolus of atropine sulfate, 0.5-1 mg, 5 minutes after the initial dose.

TABLE 20-1. Treatment of Third Degree AV Block Associated with Bradycardia and Hemodynamic Compromise

Clinical Intervention	Comments
Atropine sulfate	0.5-1 mg IV bolus; may repeat at 5 min intervals to maximum dose of 2 mg
Isoproterenol	2-10 ug/min IV infusion, titrated to desired clinical effect
Cardiac pacemaker insertion	

The maximum recommended total dose of atropine is 2 mg. If atropine fails to work, as in this case, next use isoproterenol hydrochloride, a synthetic sympathomimetic amine. Administer as a 2 to 10 ug/min IV infusion, titrated to produce the desired clinical effect. Because it is a pure β-adrenergic agonist with powerful inotropic and chronotropic properties, use with extreme caution so as not to worsen preexisting myocardial ischemia or induce additional cardiac arrhythmias.

When both atropine and isoproterenol are ineffective, the only other recourse is transport to the hospital, where definitive treatment can be undertaken with the use of an artificial cardiac pacemaker.

Field Diagnosis

- Cardiac arrhythmia with hemodynamic compromise
- Third degree AV block

Hospital Diagnosis

- Complete third degree AV block

Patient Follow-Up

Following admission to the hospital your patient was transferred to the cardiac care unit (CCU) where a pacemaker was inserted. A 12 lead electrocardiogram showed evidence of a massive inferior wall myocardial infarction; cardiac enzyme measurement also indicated that a massive infarct had taken place. On the second day in the hospital the patient developed florid pulmonary edema and became severely hypotensive. Despite aggressive measures his condition worsened. The following day he suffered full cardiopulmonary arrest and died.

Answers

1. C
    Caroline NL: Emergency Care in the Streets, 3rd ed, pp 276–286. Boston, Little, Brown & Co, 1987
    Huff J, Doernbach DP, White D: ECG Workout: Exercises In Arrhythmia Interpretation, pp 109, 234 (strip 3.90). Philadelphia, JB Lippincott, 1985
    Alpert MA: Cardiac Arrhythmias, pp 156–164. Chicago, Year Book Medical Publishers, 1980

2. B
    Caroline NL: Emergency Care in the Streets, 3rd ed, pp 252–258. Boston, Little, Brown & Co, 1987

3. C
    Alpert MA: Cardiac Arrhythmias, pp 158–164. Chicago, Year Book Medical Publishers, 1980
    Goldberger E, Wheat MW Jr: Treatment of Cardiac Emergencies, 3rd ed, pp 71–73. St Louis, CV Mosby, 1982
    American Heart Association: Standards and guidelines for cardiopulmonary resuscitation (CPR) and emergency cardiac care (ECC). JAMA 255:2905–2989, 1986

4. A
    Alpert MA: Cardiac Arrhythmias, pp 158–164. Chicago, Year Book Medical Publishers, 1980

Goldberger E, Wheat MW Jr: Treatment of Cardiac Emergencies, 3rd ed, pp 71–73. St Louis, CV Mosby, 1982

American Heart Association: Standards and guidelines for cardiopulmonary resuscitation (CPR) and emergency cardiac care (ECC). JAMA 255:2905–2989, 1986

5. E

Huff J, Doernbach DP, White D: ECG Workout: Exercises In Arrhythmia Interpretation, pp 91, 230 (strip 3.37). Philadelphia, JB Lippincott, 1985

Marriott HJL: Practical Electrocardiography, 7th ed, pp 330–332. Baltimore, Williams & Wilkins, 1983

6. B

Alpert MA: Cardiac Arrhythmias, pp 158–164. Chicago, Year Book Medical Publishers, 1980

American Heart Association: Standards and guidelines for cardiopulmonary resuscitation (CPR) and emergency cardiac care (ECC). JAMA 255:2905–2989, 1986

7. B

Caroline NL: Emergency Care in the Streets, 3rd ed, pp 276–314. Boston, Little, Brown & Co, 1987

Selected Reading

American Heart Association: Standards and guidelines for cardiopulmonary resuscitation (CPR) and emergency cardiac care (ECC). JAMA 255:2905, 1986

PEDIATRIC EMERGENCIES

21

Acute Respiratory Distress in an Infant

You and your partner respond to a report of an "infant not breathing." After a rapid response, you are led into a small apartment by two young parents who tell you that their 8-month-old child suddenly developed severe difficulty breathing and started gasping for air. Further questioning reveals that the child has no significant medical history, has not had fever, sore throat, or other medical problems recently, and has never had a similar episode before. The child has no known allergies and there is no family history of medical problems.

Rapid assessment of the patient's condition reveals a well-nourished, well-developed 8-month-old girl who appears in severe respiratory distress. Respiration appears labored, with high-pitched noises during inhalation and periodic ineffective coughs. On auscultation, breath sounds are notably diminished bilaterally. There are no signs of gross trauma. The remainder of the examination is unremarkable.

Questions

Read each question carefully, keeping in mind the context of the case at hand. Select the best answer from the choices presented.

1. The best diagnosis in this case is
   A. Laryngeal trauma
   B. Croup
   C. Foreign body obstruction
   D. Epiglottitis

2. An attempt to relieve foreign body obstruction should be made
   A. In all cases of *partial airway obstruction* and in some cases of *complete airway obstruction*
   B. In all cases of *complete airway obstruction* and in some cases of *partial airway obstruction*
   C. In all cases of *partial airway obstruction* and in all cases of *complete airway obstruction*

D. In some cases of *partial airway obstruction* and in some cases of *complete airway obstruction*

3. Use of the Heimlich maneuver (subdiaphragmatic abdominal thrusts) to help relieve foreign body obstruction is indicated in which of the following cases?
   1. An 8-month-old infant with complete airway obstruction
   2. A 2-year-old child with partial airway obstruction associated with stridor and ineffective air exchange
   3. A 6-month-old infant with partial airway obstruction associated with stridor and ineffective air exchange
   4. An 18-month-old child with complete airway obstruction

   A. 1, 2, and 3 are correct
   B. 1 and 3 are correct
   C. 2 and 4 are correct
   D. Only 4 is correct
   E. All are correct

4. Which of the following correctly describes the preferred sequence of treatment for your patient?
   A. Four back blows—four chest thrusts—open airway with head-tilt/chin-lift maneuver—inspect mouth for foreign body
   B. Four abdominal thrusts (Heimlich maneuver)—open airway with head-tilt/chin-lift maneuver—inspect mouth for foreign body
   C. Four back blows—four chest thrusts—blind sweep of mouth—head-tilt/chin-lift maneuver
   D. Four back blows—four chest thrusts—four abdominal thrusts (Heimlich maneuver)—open airway with head-tilt/chin-lift maneuver—inspect mouth for foreign body

Discussion

A young infant presents with an acute onset of severe respiratory distress. The first step in managing respiratory distress in an infant or child is to recognize its presence. The next step in management is rapidly to determine the cause of the patient's respiratory problem, which will greatly affect the type of treatment to provide. Labored respiration, ineffective cough, and stridor should alert you to the possibility of airway obstruction. Common causes of airway obstruction in the pediatric age group include

Foreign body obstruction
Infectious processes
• Croup
• Epiglottitis
• Bronchiolitis
Asthma

Certain questions may help clarify the cause of the patient's problems.

- Has the child been ill lately with fever, sore throat, cough or other flulike symptoms? If so, consider the possibility of an infectious process.
- Does the child have any medical problems? Is this the first episode of respiratory distress? Inquire about the possibility of asthma and other respiratory conditions. Also ask about any allergies, since an anaphylactic reaction may produce airway obstruction and severe respiratory distress.
- Where was the child and what was she doing when she started having difficulty breathing? Remember that foreign body obstruction is particularly common in infants and young children. If the child was eating or playing with small objects (toys, coins, peanuts) then foreign body obstruction is quite likely.

Nothing in this child's medical history suggests asthma or any other medical condition as an explanation of the present problem. Nor does the history suggest an infectious process such as croup, bronchiolitis, or epiglottitis, since there is no report of recent fever, sore throat, or cough. The acute onset of the problem, along with the physical findings, strongly suggests foreign body obstruction as the cause of this patient's problem.

Foreign body obstruction may produce either *complete* or *partial airway obstruction.* Complete airway obstruction occurs when a foreign body lodges in a portion of the respiratory tract and completely blocks the passage of air either into or out of the lungs; no air exchange is possible, and respiratory arrest and then cardiac arrest soon follow unless the obstruction is relieved. In partial airway obstruction, a foreign body lodges at some point in the airway but does not completely block air passage.

Clinically, the patient with partial airway obstruction may present in one of two ways. In some cases, the patient may still be capable of adequate air exchange; good skin color, forceful and effective coughing, and adequate breath sounds on auscultation all imply *partial airway obstruction with good air exchange.* In such a case, encourage the patient to continue coughing and rapidly transport her to a medical facility. In other cases, symptoms may include ineffective coughs, stridor, and notably diminished breath sounds on auscultation; such a case of *partial airway obstruction with poor air exchange* requires immediate treatment and should be handled as if complete airway obstruction were present.

In the present case, the patient exhibits severe respiratory distress, harsh, high-pitched inspiratory sounds (stridor), and weak ineffective coughs. A diagnosis of *partial airway obstruction with poor air exchange* is indicated. Treatment calls for immediate attempts to relieve the obstruction and facilitate air exchange. Use the Heimlich maneuver (subdiaphragmatic abdominal thrusts) for the child over 1 year of age with airway obstruction. Current recommendations call for a combination of back blows and chest compression, instead of the Heimlich maneuver, for patients under 1 year of age. In view of our patient's age (8 months), the appropriate treatment sequence includes the following:

- With the infant in a head-down position, administer four back blows between the shoulder blades with the heel of the hand.

- With the infant in a supine position and still in a head-down position, administer four chest compressions.
- Use the *head-tilt/chin-lift* maneuver to open the airway and attempt to visualize the foreign body.

> **Field Diagnosis**
> - Acute respiratory distress
> - Partial airway obstruction with poor air exchange
>
> **Hospital Diagnosis**
> - Partial airway obstruction secondary to foreign body aspiration

Patient Follow-Up

After you repeatedly attempted to relieve the obstruction, the patient finally expelled a small glass marble. Supplemental oxygen was administered, effective spontaneous respiration resumed, and the patient was transported to a medical facility for further evaluation.

Answers

1. C
2. B
3. C
4. A

See Selected Reading for source of answers in chapter 21.

Selected Reading

American Heart Association: Standards and guidelines for cardiopulmonary resuscitation (CPR) and emergency cardiac care (ECC). JAMA 255:2905, 1986

22

Cough and Fever in a Pediatric Patient

It is a rainy Sunday morning and as you and your partner, both exhausted from the busy night, pull your vehicle into the garage to try to get some rest, your dispatcher calls with a report of a sick child. Exchanging glances, you take down the necessary information and begin your response. Upon arrival, you are met by a young couple who report that their 5-year-old daughter awoke this morning with a bad cough and a high fever. Further questioning reveals that these symptoms seemed to come on suddenly; yesterday their daughter was a little tired but otherwise appeared fine. No other family members are presently ill and your patient has no significant medical history. She is taking no prescribed medications and has no reported allergies. No recent trauma is reported.

Your physical examination shows an extremely ill-looking child who is flushed, sitting in an erect position, leaning forward, and appearing in severe respiratory distress with audible stridor. Vital signs are BP (left arm, sitting) 80/60, pulse 140 full and regular, respiration 26 regular and labored, and temperature warm to touch. Head and neck examination shows no visible signs of a foreign body within the throat or oropharynx, although copious amounts of secretions are present. The tonsils appear of normal size and are without an exudate, but the pharynx is red. The trachea is midline. There is no external edema or subcutaneous emphysema in the surrounding soft tissues. Auscultation of the neck shows marked stridor. Heart and lung sounds are present but obscured. No evidence of a rash, hives, or pruritus is present. The remainder of the physical examination is unremarkable. Your patient's cardiac rhythm is that shown in Figure 22–1.

As you begin treating your patient, the parents ask whether their daughter needs to go to the hospital. They ask if you can give her some medicine and then let them treat her at home.

Questions

Read each question carefully, keeping in mind the context of the case under discussion. Select the best answer from the choices presented.

1. All of the following are signs of respiratory distress except
   A. Use of abdominal muscles to assist with inhalation
   B. Nasal flaring

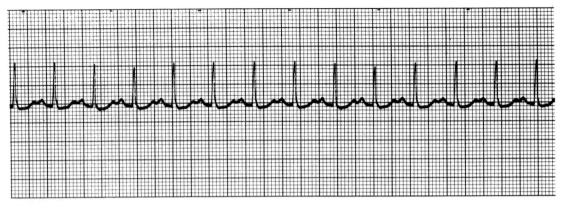

FIGURE 22-1. Lead II EKG recorded shortly after arrival at the scene.

   C. Use of accessory muscles (sternocleidomastoid and scalene muscles)
   D. Retraction of intercostal muscles during inhalation

2. The abnormal respiratory stridor that was present in your patient is best described as a
   A. Low-pitched rattling sound present during inspiration
   B. High-pitched sound with a musical quality present both on inspiration and expiration
   C. Low-pitched sound of a crackling or bubbling nature and present primarily on inspiration
   D. High-pitched sound with a harsh quality present on inhalation

3. Which of the following sets of values represent normal vital signs in a 6-year-old female patient such as yours?
   A. BP 120/80, pulse 110/min, respiration 18/min
   B. BP 100/88, pulse 135/min, respiration 20/min
   C. BP 106/66, pulse 100/min, respiration 18/min
   D. BP 80/84, pulse 75/min, respiration 16/min
   E. BP 92/60, pulse 84/min, respiration 22/min

4. Upper airway obstruction is associated with which of the following abnormal respiratory sounds?
   A. Wheezing and rhonchi
   B. Stridor and snoring
   C. Rales and rhonchi
   D. Snoring and rhonchi
   E. Rales and wheezing

5. In a pediatric patient with acute respiratory distress, all of the following should be considered in the differential diagnosis except
   A. Foreign body obstruction

B. Chronic obstructive pulmonary disease
C. Bronchiolitis
D. Asthma
E. Laryngotracheobronchitis
F. Epiglottitis

6. Regarding bronchiolitis, all of the following statements are true except
   A. It is a condition characterized by inflammation of the bronchioles
   B. It is most common in children between the ages of 6 and 10
   C. It often presents with expiratory wheezing
   D. It is caused by a virus

7. All of the following statements regarding croup are true except
   A. It is also called laryngotracheobronchitis
   B. It is a viral infection of the upper airways
   C. It is most common in children between 4 and 6 years of age
   D. It is often associated with hoarseness and a high-pitched stridor ("seal bark")

8. All of the following statements about epiglottitis are true except
   A. It is a bacterial infection of the epiglottis
   B. It normally has a gradual and progressive onset
   C. It is most common in children greater than 3 years of age
   D. It is often associated with a high-pitched stridor

9. Regarding the acute asthmatic attack, all of the following statements are true except
   A. It may be seen in young children as well as adults
   B. It is characterized by respiratory wheezing
   C. It is due to widespread alveolar destruction
   D. The chest often yields a hyperresonant note when percussed

10. Which of the following pairs correctly links a medical condition with the age range in which it most commonly occurs?
    A. Asthma—50 to 60 years of age
    B. Croup—4 to 6 years of age
    C. Epiglottitis—over 4 years of age
    D. Bronchiolitis—3 to 6 years of age

11. High fever, copious oropharyngeal secretions, and your patient's age (5 years) point most strongly to a diagnosis of
    A. Asthma
    B. Foreign body obstruction
    C. Epiglottitis
    D. Bronchiolitis
    E. Croup

12. Treatment should include all of the following except
    A. Administration of humidified oxygen
    B. Visualization of the epiglottis and surrounding area
    C. Placement in a position of comfort
    D. Rapid transport
    E. Establishment of an intravenous line with D5/W, if easily accomplished

13. The most feared complication associated with your patient's condition is
    A. Complete airway obstruction
    B. Aspiration pneumonia
    C. Dehydration
    D. Cardiac arrhythmias

14. Your patient's cardiac rhythm (Figure 22-1) is best classified as
    A. Sinus bradycardia
    B. Normal sinus rhythm
    C. Sinus tachycardia
    D. Ventricular tachycardia

Discussion

You are presented with a 5-year-old girl who appears extremely ill and is in severe respiratory distress. Correct definition of the patient's problem requires an understanding of both the normal anatomy of the respiratory system and of various conditions that can induce the acute onset of respiratory distress in a pediatric patient.

For purposes of discussion, the respiratory system can be divided into several anatomically distinct regions, including the pharynx, larynx, trachea, bronchi, and the terminal portions of the respiratory tree, which are known as the bronchioles and which in turn lead into the alveoli. The pharynx is in contact with both the nasal and oral cavities and extends vertically to the larynx. A flap of tissue known as the epiglottis guards the entrance from the pharynx into the larynx. The larynx is a tubular structure that extends vertically to the level of the sixth cervical vertebra, where the cricoid cartilages mark the entrance into the trachea. The trachea extends approximately 12 cm (in the adult) to the level of the fifth thoracic vertebra, where it bifurcates into right and left mainstem bronchi. The bronchi branch into the small-diameter conducting airways known as bronchioles. Below the bronchioles are the alveoli, where the actual process of gas exchange takes place.

The above discussion contains several points of clinical importance. First, because the epiglottis serves as the entrance where air passes from the pharynx into the larynx and finally into the lungs, any condition that causes the epiglottis to obstruct this entrance also obstructs the passage of air, resulting in impaired gas exchange and respiratory distress. Second, the finding of hoarseness in a patient suggests laryngeal involvement, since the vocal cords are located in the larynx.

A final point of clinical importance involves the division of the trachea into the right and left mainstem bronchi. The left bronchus branches off the trachea at a moderately sharp angle, but the right bronchus branches off at much less of an angle and extends more vertically. Thus foreign body obstruction is more likely to involve the right mainstem bronchus. For the same reason, an endotracheal tube passed too far will wind up in the right bronchus.

The next step is to consider the conditions that can account for the acute onset of respiratory distress in a pediatric patient. Possibilities include traumatic injury, burns or inhalational injury, bronchospastic diseases such as asthma, foreign body obstruction of the airway, anaphylactic reactions, and infectious diseases that produce airway obstruction. Trauma, burns, and inhalational injury to the respiratory system are unlikely in the present case, since the parents report no recently-sustained injury, accident, or smoke inhalation. An anaphylactic reaction is similarly unlikely, since the parent's indicate that their daughter has no known allergies and since you find no rash, hives, or pruritus (itching). Foreign body obstruction, although a possibility, is not likely since the patient's symptoms seemed to come on shortly after she woke up and before she could ingest any food or other material.

The remaining possible causes include asthma and infectious disease. According to the parents, the patient has no history of medical problems (such as asthma). This fact and the associated fever and general malaise exhibited by your patient suggest that the problem is of an infectious nature. Although there are a myriad of infectious diseases that may produce respiratory distress, three conditions of particular importance in pediatric patients are bronchiolitis, laryngotracheobronchitis, and acute epiglottitis.

Bronchiolitis is a condition characterized by inflammation of the small airway passages, specifically the bronchioles (see "Acute Bronchiolitis"). It is usually of viral origin and is most common in children under 2 years of age. It frequently presents a picture similar to asthma, including respiratory difficulty and expiratory wheezing.

Acute Bronchiolitis

AGE: Usually found in children less than 2 years of age with a peak incidence at 6 months of age

ETIOLOGY: An infectious process of viral etiology; commonly due to respiratory syncytial virus, parainfluenza virus, and adenoviruses

PATHOPHYSIOLOGY: Hallmark is obstruction of the bronchioles secondary to edema and mucous plugging

CLINICAL FEATURES

- Recent history of mild upper respiratory tract infection
- Tachypnea
- Cyanosis
- Nasal flaring
- Use of accessory muscles
- Diffuse rales and wheezing
- Prolonged expiration

(continued)

Other Conditions To Consider

- Asthma
- Foreign body obstruction
- Epiglottitis
- Laryngotracheobronchitis

Field Treatment

- Administer humidified oxygen
- Place in position of comfort
- Monitor cardiac rhythm and vital signs
- Transport to hospital
- Options (if advised by medical control):

  1. Administer epinephrine 1:1,000, 0.01 mg/kg subcutaneously repeated in 20–30 minutes if needed
  2. Have intubation materials ready in case they are needed

Laryngotracheobronchitis, also known as croup, involves inflammation of the subglottic tissue. Inflammation is located just below the epiglottis in the initial part of the larynx and extends a variable distance downward to the trachea and in some cases to the bronchiolar system (see "Laryngotracheobronchitis"). It is of viral origin and is most common in children between 6 months and 4 years of age. More frequent in boys than girls, it occurs with a peak incidence during the late fall. Classically, there is an acute onset of respiratory distress with hoarseness, cough, and a high-pitched inspiratory stridor that many have likened to a "seal bark."

Laryngotracheobronchitis

AGE: Most common in children between the ages of 6 months and 4 years of age

ETIOLOGY: An infectious process of viral etiology

PATHOPHYSIOLOGY: Starts as an upper airway infection and then travels downward to involve the bronchi and bronchioles.

Clinical Features

Cough
Stridor
Inspiratory stridor
Prolonged expiratory phase
Agitation and irritability
Pyrexia
Diminished breath sounds
Diffuse rhonchi and rales
Marked respiratory distress
- Nasal flaring
- Tracheal tugging
- Use of accessory muscles

Cyanosis
Tachycardia
Tachypnea

(continued)

OTHER CONDITIONS TO CONSIDER

Epiglottitis
Bronchiolitis
Foreign body obstruction
Asthma

FIELD TREATMENT

Administer humidified oxygen
Place in position of comfort
Transport to hospital
Monitor cardiac rhythm and vital signs
Options (if advised by medical control):
- Establish IV access
- Racemic epinephrine (Vasonephrin), 0.5 ml in 2.5 ml saline via nebulization

---

Acute epiglottitis is a bacterial infection that causes inflammation of the epiglottis. Edema and swelling result (see "Epiglottitis"). It is most common in children between the ages of 4 and 7 years and often has an acute onset with rapid progression. It is frequently associated with high fever and copious oropharyngeal secretions. Severe respiratory distress, sitting in an erect, forward-leaning posture, and an audible inspiratory stridor are common. This is a true medical emergency requiring prompt recognition and transport because the swollen cherry red epiglottis may completely obstruct the airway.

Epiglottitis

AGE: Most common in children between the ages of 4 and 7 years of age

ETIOLOGY: An infectious process of bacterial etiology generally caused by *Hemophilus influenza,* type b

PATHOPHYSIOLOGY: Marked inflammation of the epiglottis (*i.e.,* "cherry red epiglottis") and surrounding tissues

CLINICAL FEATURES

Abrupt onset
Fever
Drooling
Aphonia
Inspiratory stridor
Hoarseness
Cough
Irritability
Marked respiratory distress
- Nasal flaring
- Tracheal tugging
- Use of accessory muscles
- Sternal retractions
Abnormal breath sounds
Tachycardia
Tachypnea
Diaphoresis

(continued)

FIELD TREATMENT

Administer humidified oxygen
Establish IV access if feasible
Place in position of comfort
Secure rapid transport

> DO NOT ATTEMPT TO VISUALIZE THE EPIGLOTTIS OR PERFORM ANY MANIPULATIONS OF THE AIRWAY SINCE SEVERE LARYNGOSPASM MAY ENSUE

Several key points are helpful in arriving at a diagnosis in this case. The acute onset and rapid progression of the patient's condition, and the presence of a high fever and severe respiratory distress, are consistent with the symptoms of epiglottitis. The age of your patient is also in favor of a diagnosis of epiglottitis since both bronchiolitis and laryngotracheobronchitis tend to occur in younger patients. Lastly, the patient's copious oropharyngeal secretions and assumption of an erect and forward-leaning posture also point to acute epiglottitis. Thus, a reasonable working field diagnosis for this patient is severe respiratory distress secondary to acute bacterial epiglottitis.

Treatment should involve monitoring vital signs and cardiac rhythm, administration of humidified oxygen, establishment of an intravenous line, and rapid transport. It is extremely important to avoid any maneuver or procedure that might precipitate increased swelling or laryngospasm and cause complete airway obstruction. Attempts to visualize the patient's throat with a laryngoscope or even a simple tongue depressor should be strictly avoided because life-threatening laryngospasm may result.

Field Diagnosis
- Acute bacterial epiglottitis

Hospital Diagnosis
- Acute bacterial epiglottitis

Patient Follow-Up

Following transport to the emergency room, the patient continued to show serious clinical deterioration. Careful assessment, including a lateral radiograph (Figure 22-2), revealed a severely inflamed epiglottis. Acute bacterial epiglottitis was diagnosed. A decision was made to perform a tracheotomy. After intensive treatment with antibiotics and respiratory support, your patient recovered and was discharged from the hospital.

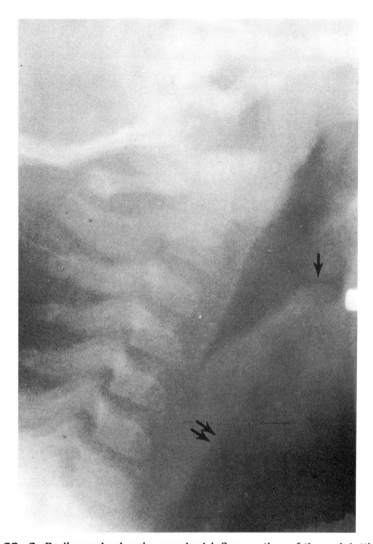

FIGURE 22-2. Radiograph showing marked inflammation of the epiglottis. Single arrow shows epiglottic swelling while the double arrow points to a normal subglottic airway. (Burton GG, Gee GN, Hodgkin JE [eds]: Respiratory Care: A Guide to Clinical Practice, 2nd ed, p 777. Philadelphia, JB Lippincott, 1984)

Answers

1. A

    Caroline NL: Emergency Care in the Streets, 3rd ed, p 180. Boston, Little, Brown & Co, 1987

    Grant HD, Murray RH Jr, Bergeron JD: Emergency Care, 4th ed, p 87. Englewood Cliffs, NJ, Prentice-Hall, 1986

2. D

    Caroline NL: Emergency Care in the Streets, 3rd ed, p 181. Boston, Little, Brown & Co, 1987

    American Academy of Orthopaedic Surgeons: Emergency Care and Transportation of the Sick and Injured, 4th ed, p 620. Menasha, WI, George Banta Co, 1987

3. E

Caroline NL: Emergency Care in the Streets, 3rd ed, p 519. Boston, Little, Brown & Co, 1987

4. B

Caroline NL: Emergency Care in the Streets, 3rd ed, p 181. Boston, Little, Brown & Co, 1987

Caroline NL: Emergency Medical Treatment: A Text for EMT-As and EMT-Intermediates, 2nd ed, p 199. Boston, Little, Brown & Co, 1987

5. B

Caroline NL: Emergency Care in the Streets, 3rd ed, pp 507–515. Boston, Little, Brown & Co, 1987

Caroline NL: Emergency Medical Treatment: A Text for EMT-As and EMT-Intermediates, 2nd ed, pp 505–508. Boston, Little, Brown & Co, 1987

Grant HD, Murray RH Jr, Bergeron JD: Emergency Care, 4th ed, pp 382–383. Englewood Cliffs, NJ, Prentice-Hall, 1986

6. B

Caroline NL: Emergency Care in the Streets, 3rd ed, pp 512–513. Boston, Little, Brown & Co, 1987

Stern RC: Acute bronchiolitis. In Behrman RE, Vaughan VC III, Nelson WC: Textbook of Pediatrics, 12th ed. Philadelphia, WB Saunders, 1983

7. C

Caroline NL: Emergency Care in the Streets, 3rd ed, pp 513–514. Boston, Little, Brown & Co, 1987

Grant HD, Murray RH Jr, Bergeron JD: Emergency Care, 4th ed, p 382. Englewood Cliffs, NJ, Prentice-Hall, 1986

Stern RC: Acute infections of the larynx and trachea. In Behrman RE, Vaughan VC III, Nelson WC: Textbook of Pediatrics, 12th ed. Philadelphia, WB Saunders, 1983

8. B

Grant HD, Murray RH Jr, Bergeron JD: Emergency Care, 4th ed, p 382. New Jersey, Prentice-Hall, 1986

Caroline NL: Emergency Care in the Streets, 3rd ed, pp 514–515. Boston, Little, Brown & Co, 1987

Caroline NL: Emergency Medical Treatment: A Text for EMT-As and EMT-Intermediates, 2nd ed, pp 507–589. Boston, Little, Brown & Co, 1987

Stern RC: Acute infections of the larynx and trachea. In Behrman RE, Vaughan VC III, Nelson WC: Textbook of Pediatrics, 12th ed. Philadelphia, WB Saunders, 1983

9. C

Caroline NL: Emergency Care in the Streets, 3rd ed, pp 510–511. Boston, Little, Brown & Co, 1987

Stern RC: Bronchial asthma. In Behrman RE, Vaughan VC III, Nelson WC: Textbook of Pediatrics, 12th ed. Philadelphia, WB Saunders, 1983

10. C

Caroline NL: Emergency Care in the Streets, 3rd ed, p 514. Boston, Little, Brown & Co, 1987

11. C

Caroline NL: Emergency Care in the Streets, 3rd ed, pp 514–515. Boston, Little, Brown & Co, 1987

Grant HD, Murray RH Jr, Bergeron JD: Emergency Care, 4th ed, p 382. Englewood Cliffs, NJ, Prentice-Hall, 1986

Stern RC: Acute infections of the larynx and trachea. In Behrman RE, Vaughan VC III, Nelson WC: Textbook of Pediatrics, 12th ed. Philadelphia, WB Saunders, 1983

12. B

Caroline NL: Emergency Care in the Streets, 3rd ed, pp 514–515. Boston, Little, Brown & Co, 1987

Grant HD, Murray RH Jr, Bergeron JD: Emergency Care, 4th ed, p 382. Englewood Cliffs, NJ, Prentice-Hall, 1986

Stern RC: Acute infections of the larynx and trachea. In Behrman RE, Vaughan VC III, Nelson WC: Textbook of Pediatrics, 12th ed. Philadelphia, WB Saunders, 1983

13. A

Grant HD, Murray RH Jr, Bergeron JD: Emergency Care, 4th ed, p 382. Englewood Cliffs, NJ, Prentice-Hall, 1986

Stern RC: Acute infections of the larynx and trachea. In Behrman RE, Vaughan VC III, Nelson WC: Textbook of Pediatrics, 12th ed. Philadelphia, WB Saunders, 1983

14. C

Huff J, Doernbach DP, White RD: ECG Workout: Exercises In Arrhythmia Interpretation, pp 16, 214 (strip 1.33). Philadelphia, JB Lippincott, 1985

Caroline NL: Emergency Care in the Streets, 3rd ed, p 287. Boston, Little, Brown & Co, 1987

Selected Reading

Diaz JH, Lockhart CH: Early diagnosis and airway management of acute epiglottitis in children. South Med J 75:399, 1982

Stern RC: Acute infections of the larynx and trachea. In Behrman RE, Vaughan VC III, Nelson WC: Textbook of Pediatrics, 12th ed. Philadelphia, WB Saunders, 1983

Tintinalli J: Respiratory stridor in young children. JACEP 5:195, 1976

23

Cardiopulmonary Arrest in a Pediatric Patient

You and your partner respond to a call to aid a "child not breathing." Upon arrival, you are met by the police who quickly guide you inside the house. You are met by a young couple, both of whom are frantic and in tears. They inform you that they heard a soft cry from their child's room, and after coming in to investigate, found their 18-month-old infant unresponsive in her crib. The child's medical history is significant only for premature birth at 7½ months and a recent upper respiratory tract infection.

Questions

Read each question carefully, keeping in mind the context of the case under discussion. Select the best answer from the choices presented.

1. Common causes of cardiac arrest in the pediatric age group include all the following except
   A. Acquired heart disease
   B. Injury
   C. Foreign body obstruction
   D. Infection

2. The correct sequence of treatment when approaching a child in cardiopulmonary arrest is
   1. Confirm unresponsiveness
   2. Administer cardiac compressions
   3. Check for breathing
   4. Open airway
   5. Check for pulse
   6. Administer artificial ventilation

   A. 3, 1, 5, 4, 6, 2
   B. 1, 3, 4, 5, 6, 2
   C. 1, 4, 3, 6, 5, 2

D. 4, 3, 1, 6, 5, 2
E. 3, 5, 2, 6, 4, 1

3. Accepted means of establishing an airway in your patient include
   A. Head-tilt/chin-lift or jaw thrust
   B. Neck hyperextension or head-tilt/neck-lift
   C. Head-tilt/chin-lift or neck hyperextension
   D. Jaw thrust or neck hyperextension

4. In cases of suspected cervical injury the preferred means of establishing an airway is
   A. Head-tilt/chin-lift
   B. Neck hyperextension
   C. Jaw thrust
   D. Neck flexion

5. Following your initial assessment the child is unconscious, unresponsive to verbal or painful stimuli, and without spontaneous respiration. Rescue breathing is initiated by administering
   A. Four breaths in rapid succession
   B. Two slow breaths
   C. One large breath
   D. Three breaths in rapid succession

6. The preferred site for checking for the presence of a pulse in your patient is the
   A. Brachial artery
   B. Carotid artery
   C. Radial artery
   D. Apical pulse

7. Rescue breathing is correctly carried out at a rate of
   A. 20/min for an infant—15/min for a child
   B. 10/min for a child—20/min for an infant
   C. 20/min for a child—10/min for an infant
   D. 40/min for an infant—20/min for a child

8. Chest compressions are best carried out in the infant using
   A. Two or three fingers, to a depth of 1.3–2.5 cm
   B. The heel of one hand, to a depth of 2.5–3.8 cm
   C. Two or three fingers, to a depth of 2.5–3.8 cm
   D. The heel of one hand, to a depth of 1.3–2.5 cm

9. The correct compression to ventilation ratio when performing cardiopulmonary resuscitation (CPR) is
   A. 5:1 in the infant—5:1 in the child
   B. 15:2 in the infant—5:1 in the child

C. 5:1 in the infant—15:2 in the child
D. 12:3 in the infant—15:3 in the child
E. 15:2 in the infant—15:2 in the child

10. Following initiation of CPR in your patient, respiration and pulse should first be reassessed after
    A. 5 minutes of compressions and ventilation
    B. 10 seconds of compressions and ventilation
    C. 1 minute of compressions and ventilation
    D. 3 minutes of compressions and ventilation

Discussion

Although the present scenario is straightforward, it illustrates a vital area of prehospital paramedic care, management of cardiopulmonary arrest in the pediatric patient. Although the underlying principles for treating pediatric patients are in many ways similar to those used for treating adults, there are important differences that must be appreciated.

While cardiac arrest in adults is frequently of cardiac origin, the same does not hold true in the pediatric age group. Cardiac arrest in infants and children frequently stems from noncardiac conditions, and is usually secondary to a variety of conditions that may result in severe hypoxemia (see "Etiology of Cardiopulmonary Arrest in Pediatric Patients").

Etiology of Cardiopulmonary Arrest in Pediatric Patients

Infection
- Epiglottitis
- Laryngotracheobronchitis
- Bronchiolitis

Trauma
- Motor vehicle accidents
- Burns
- Child abuse
- Drowning

Foreign body obstruction
Sudden infant death syndrome
Ingestion of toxic agents

When dealing with the pediatric patient in suspected cardiopulmonary arrest a systematic approach is essential (see "Management of Pediatric Cardiopulmonary Arrest"). First, rapidly assess the degree of injury and determine if the patient is unconscious. Gently tapping the patient, or in the case of an infant, flicking your finger against the soles of the feet, are good means of roughly determining the level of consciousness. The next step is to ensure that adequate help is available; if additional assistance will be needed, request that the police, parents, neighbors, or whoever else is present summon the appropriate assistance. Also, the paramedic

Management of Pediatric Cardiopulmonary Arrest

- Establish unresponsiveness
- Obtain necessary help
- Position patient
- Ensure patent airway
- Determine adequacy of breathing
- Administer artificial ventilation
- Check for presence of a pulse
- Administer external chest compressions
- Reassess patient after 1 min

should ensure that a flat, hard surface is available in the event that cardiopulmonary resuscitation (CPR) is necessary.

Once unresponsiveness has been established, appropriate help summoned, and the patient correctly positioned, the next step is to *ensure an open airway*. The two recommended techniques for ensuring an open airway are the head-tilt/chin-lift maneuver (see "Technique for Performing the Head-Tilt/Chin-Lift Maneuver")

Technique for Performing the Head-Tilt/Chin-Lift Maneuver

- Place hand nearest the patient's head on her forehead.
- Gently exert pressure to tilt the head back, making sure not to hyperextend.
- With the remaining hand, exert upwards traction just below the lower jaw in order to elevate the chin, using all fingers except the thumb.

> THE HEAD-TILT MANEUVER SHOULD NOT BE USED IF CERVICAL SPINE INJURY IS SUSPECTED

and the jaw-thrust maneuver. In the majority of cases, the former procedure is preferred, but in cases of suspected cervical spine injury, the latter technique is advantageous. Once an open airway has been ensured, assess the extent of the patient's spontaneous respiration, using the motto "look, listen, and feel." Place your ear above the patient's mouth and direct your eyes toward the patient's feet. Look for respiratory movements of the chest and abdomen, listen for exhaled air, and try to feel any exhaled air as it flows from the patient's mouth. If spontaneous ventilation is present, maintain the airway, administer supplemental oxygen (if needed), and monitor the patient carefully.

If no spontaneous ventilation is detected, then administer artificial ventilatory support. Current recommendations call for administering *two slow breaths* at a volume sufficient to cause the patient's chest to rise and fall. Following the initial two breaths, assess for the presence or absence of a pulse. The best means of doing this depends on the age of the patient. In patients over 1 year of age, assessing the pulse by palpating the carotid artery is recommended. In patients under 1 year of age, this method may not be feasible; current recommendations call for assessing the pulse by palpating the brachial artery. If no pulse is palpable, proceed with external cardiac compressions accompanied by artificial ventilatory support.

TABLE 23-1. External Chest Compressions for the Pediatric Patient

	Infant	Child
PATIENT POSITION	Supine on hard surface	Supine on hard surface
LOCATION	A distance the width of 1 finger below imaginary line connecting nipples; directly over sternum	Over lower half of sternum
USE FOR COMPRESSION	2 or 3 fingers	Heel of one hand
DEPTH OF COMPRESSIONS	0.5–1 in (1.3–2.5 cm)	1–1.5 in (2.5–3.8 cm)
COMPRESSION RATE	100/min	80/min
RATIO OF COMPRESSIONS TO VENTILATION	5:1	5:1

Deliver external chest compressions with the patient lying supine on a hard surface (Table 23-1). For infants, compressions should be administered at a distance the width of one finger below an imaginary line connecting the nipples. Use two or three fingers and compress the sternum to a depth of 0.5 to 1 inch (1.3–2.5 cm). Ideally, compressions should be at a rate of not less than 100 per minute. For children under 8 years of age, administer compressions over the lower half of the sternum, using the heel of one hand to depress the sternum 1 to 1.5 inches (2.5–3.8 cm). A rate of 80 to 100 compressions per minute is ideal. Regardless of the age of the patient, compressions should be delivered in a smooth fashion, avoiding jerky movement and ensuring adequate time for the chest to return to its normal position between compressions.

Alternating rescue breathing with external chest compressions is vital for successful CPR. For both infants and children a compression to ventilation ratio of 5:1 should be maintained. Respirations should be delivered at a rate of 20 per minute (1 every 3 seconds) for infants and 15 per minute (1 every 4 seconds) for children.

Field Diagnosis
- Cardiopulmonary arrest

Hospital Diagnosis
- Cardiopulmonary arrest, etiology unknown

Patient Follow-Up

The patient was rapidly transported to the hospital emergency room with BLS and ACLS in progress. Although medical personnel made aggressive attempts at resuscitation both in the field and in the hospital, the patient was pronounced dead 1 hour after arriving at the hospital.

Answers

1. A
2. C
3. A
4. C
5. B
6. B
7. A
8. A
9. A
10. C

See Selected Reading, American Heart Association article, for source of answers in chapter 23.

Selected Reading

American Heart Association: Standards and guidelines for cardiopulmonary resuscitation (CPR) and emergency cardiac care (ECC). JAMA 255:2905 (see pp 2954–2958), 1986

Grauer K, Cavallaro D: ACLS: Certification Preparation and a Comprehensive Review, 2nd ed. St Louis, CV Mosby, 1987

Seidel JS, Hornbein M, Yoshiyama K et al: Emergency medical services and the pediatric patient: Are the needs being met? Pediatrics 73:769, 1987

Ludwig S, Kettrick RG, Parker M: Pediatric cardiopulmonary resuscitation. Clin Pediatr 23:71, 1984

24

Upper Extremity Injury in a 5-Year-Old Boy

You and your partner respond to a report of an "injured child." It is a cold and rainy day and, after advising a delayed arrival time due to poor road conditions, you begin your response. Arriving in front of a large apartment complex, you are directed to a tenth floor apartment by the police. Inside, the parents relate that their 5-year-old child was playing outside with his friends when he "had a fight and hurt his arm." They indicate that their son has no significant past medical history and takes no medications, and insist he has never required hospitalization.

During physical examination, you find a quiet and somewhat reserved 5-year-old boy who weighs approximately 35 pounds. Vital signs are BP 88/62, pulse 125, and respiration 26. Examination of the head and neck is unremarkable; the conjunctiva are pink and nonicteric and the trachea appears midline. The thorax appears without deformity, respiratory excursion is symmetrical, and breath sounds are clear bilaterally. There is moderate to severe tenderness to palpation over the upper right rib cage. The abdomen is flat and nondistended; a left subcostal surgical scar is apparent, as are several small areas of ecchymosis. Bowel sounds are present. On palpation there is some voluntary guarding although the patient denies any pain. Examination of the extremities reveals marked deformity, angulation, and swelling over the lower portion of the right arm. Distal pulses are present in the affected extremity, as are sensation and some spontaneous movement. The remaining extremities are unremarkable and without signs of injury. Neurologically, the patient appears alert and oriented, and there are no focal findings. The remainder of the examination is unremarkable except for some bruises over the lower back.

Vital signs repeated 10 minutes after arrival show BP 92/64, pulse 120, and respiration 28; orthostatic changes are absent. Cardiac monitoring and treatment are initiated (Figure 24–1).

Questions

Read each question carefully, keeping in mind the context of the case under discussion. Select the best answer from the choices presented.

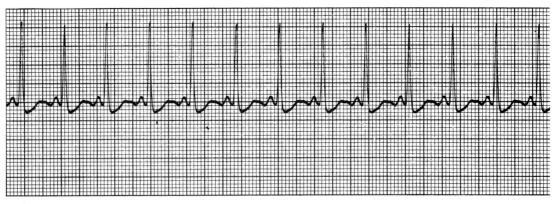

FIGURE 24-1. Lead II EKG recorded shortly after arrival at the scene.

1. Which, if any, of your patient's initial vital signs (BP 88/62, pulse 125, respiration 26) are outside of the normal range?
    1. Diastolic blood pressure
    2. Systolic blood pressure
    3. Pulse
    4. Respiration

    A. 1, 2, and 3 are correct
    B. 1 and 3 are correct
    C. 2 and 4 are correct
    D. All of the above are correct
    E. None of the above are correct

2. Swelling, deformity, and angulation of the upper right extremity are most consistent with
    A. Fracture of the radius
    B. Superficial cellulitis
    C. Fracture of the humerus
    D. Osteoporosis

3. Your patient's electrocardiogram is best interpreted as
    A. Normal sinus rhythm
    B. Atrial fibrillation
    C. Sinus tachycardia
    D. Third degree AV block

4. Additional concerns about your patient should include the possibility of
    1. Acute myocardial infarction
    2. Child abuse
    3. Significant intraabdominal hemorrhage
    4. Rib fracture

A. 1, 2, and 3 are correct
B. 1 and 3 are correct
C. 2 and 4 are correct
D. Only 4 is correct
E. All of the above are correct

5. Proper management of your patient's extremity injury should include application of
   A. A traction splint (Thomas splint)
   B. MAST
   C. A rigid splint (padded board splint)
   D. A pillow splint

Discussion

The patient presents with both an acute medical problem and evidence of child abuse. Child abuse is a frequent, although often overlooked, condition. It is extremely important that the paramedic be well versed at recognizing and reporting suspected cases of abuse (see "Child Abuse").

Child Abuse

Types of Child Abuse

- Physical abuse
- Sexual abuse
- Psychological abuse
- Neglect

Epidemiology

- 500,000–1,000,000 cases of child abuse each year
- 1,000–4,000 deaths each year due to child abuse
- 10% of all injuries in children under 5 who are seen in the emergency room are the result of child abuse

Clinical Features

- Unexplained injuries
- Inconsistencies between history and physical findings
- Failure to thrive
- Bruises, abrasions, and lacerations
- Evidence of old burns

Treatment

- Treat any acute medical problems
- Document completely all findings and information provided
- Do not discuss the possibility of child abuse with the child's family
- Convey your suspicions of child abuse to the emergency room physician
- If appropriate contact local authorities

Child abuse takes many different forms; physical abuse, sexual abuse, and neglect are only a few of the more common patterns that may be encountered. The magnitude of this problem is reflected in several startling statistics. One to two percent of all children in the United States suffer from some form of abuse during childhood. Furthermore, up to 10% of children under the age of 5 who are seen in the emergency room for physical injuries are victims of child abuse. In cases of physical abuse the perpetrator is, in the overwhelming majority of cases, a family member. It is also important to be aware that child abuse has no socioeconomic boundaries; it occurs among the rich and the poor, the educated and the uneducated, the religious and the nonreligious.

The clinical features of child abuse are often subtle and nonspecific. A good history may provide the first clue to the possibility of child abuse. There are often obvious discrepancies between the parents' report and the physical examination results, as in the present case. The parents' story that their child was "outside playing" when he "had a fight with his friend and hurt his arm" should immediately raise suspicion. The physical findings suggest a major fracture to the right humerus, an injury that could only be caused by substantial trauma. It should be obvious that the patient did far more than "hurt his arm," and it is certainly questionable whether a fight with another small child could produce an injury of this magnitude. Other inconsistencies are also present; although the parents deny any medical history or hospitalizations, the physical examination reveals a left subcostal surgical scar. Although the above information certainly does not prove child abuse, it definitely raises it as a question that needs further clarification.

The physical examination may alert you to the possibility of child abuse. Bruises and burns are particularly common in physically abused children and should be carefully noted, especially when they are multiple and without adequate explanation, and are found incidentally or in unusual places. Your patient has several unexplained bruises over the lower back and ecchymotic areas over the abdomen, all of which are certainly suspicious findings. The pain that is elicited over the rib cage during routine palpation is also unexplained. The possibility of a trauma-induced rib fracture must be entertained. Taken in total, the physical findings are troublesome and are not adequately explained. The possibility of physical abuse must be recognized.

Treatment of this patient, as with all cases of potential child abuse, requires managing any acute medical problems and transporting him to a medical facility, as well as reporting your suspicions to the appropriate authority. In this case, the most immediate problem is the upper extremity. The findings of pain, deformity, and angulation suggest an underlying fracture of the humerus. Treatment should involve gentle traction and immobilization with a rigid splint. Frequent monitoring of vital signs and checking for the presence of a distal pulse are also indicated.

Addressing the possibility of child abuse is somewhat more difficult. Carefully and completely document any and all observed injuries, as well as other pertinent findings. Do not attempt to confront the parents; instead, transport the patient to a medical facility for further evaluation, treatment, and protection. Convey to the hospital physician your suspicions of child abuse. Even if you fear you will not be taken seriously or that the matter will not be adequately addressed, you have a moral, if not legal, obligation to report your suspicions to the appropriate authorities.

Field Diagnosis

- Fracture of right humerus
- Possible rib fracture
- Unexplained soft-tissue injuries

Hospital Diagnosis

- Fracture of right humerus
- Rib fracture
- Child abuse

Patient Follow-Up

Your patient was evaluated in the emergency room and diagnosed as having sustained a spiral fracture to the distal portion of the right humerus, in addition to a fracture of the fourth rib on the right side. The emergency room staff were concerned about the possibility of child abuse and admitted the patient for observation. The authorities were notified, and a complete investigation uncovered a long history of child abuse with multiple hospital admissions.

Answers

1. E

    Caroline NL: Emergency Care in the Streets, 3rd ed, p 518. Boston, Little, Brown & Co, 1987

    Behrman RE, Vaughan VC III, Nelson WC: Textbook of Pediatrics, 12th ed, pp 1100–1102. Philadelphia, WB Saunders, 1983

    Grant HD, Murray RH Jr, Bergeron JD: Emergency Care, 4th ed, p 376. Englewood Cliffs, NJ, Prentice-Hall, 1986

2. C

    American Academy of Orthopaedic Surgeons: Emergency Care and Transportation of the Sick and Injured, 4th ed, pp 171–172. Menasha, WI, George Banta Co, 1987

    Grant HD, Murray RH Jr, Bergeron JD: Emergency Care, 4th ed, pp 208, 212. Englewood Cliffs, NJ, Prentice-Hall, 1986

    Caroline NL: Emergency Care in the Streets, 3rd ed, pp 407–410. Boston, Little, Brown & Co, 1987

3. A

    Grauer K, Cavallaro D: ACLS: Certification Preparation and a Comprehensive Review, 2nd ed, p 418. St Louis, CV Mosby, 1987

    Garson A: The Electrocardiogram in Infants and Children: A Systematic Approach. Philadelphia, Lea & Febiger, 1983

4. C

    Behrman RE, Vaughan VC III, Nelson WC: Textbook of Pediatrics, 12th ed, pp 99–102. Philadelphia, WB Saunders, 1983

    Caroline NL: Emergency Care in the Streets, 3rd ed, pp 516–518. Boston, Little, Brown & Co, 1987

    Grant HD, Murray RH Jr, Bergeron JD: Emergency Care, 4th ed, pp 379–381. Englewood Cliffs, NJ, Prentice-Hall, 1986

5. C

    American Academy of Orthopaedic Surgeons: Emergency Care and Transportation of the Sick and Injured, 4th ed. pp 198–199. Menasha, WI, George Banta Co, 1987

Selected Reading

Armstrong K, Cantwell HB, Garbarino J, Hunner R et al: Child abuse: The EMS response. J Emerg Care Trans 15:11, 1986

Behrman RE, Vaughan III VC, Nelson WC: Textbook of Pediatrics, 12th ed. pp 99–105. Philadelphia, WB Saunders, 1983

Kempe CH, Helfer RE (eds): The Battered Child, 3rd ed. Chicago, University of Chicago Press, 1980

25

A 3-Year-Old Child with Sudden Shortness of Breath

You are dispatched to a small house on the outskirts of town to help a "child with difficulty breathing." After a rapid response you quickly secure the vehicle and proceed into the house, where a young couple directs you into the living room. Their 3-year-old daughter is diaphoretic and in obvious respiratory distress. The parents relate that she has had several identical episodes in the past, with the first occurring when she was 18 months old. They inform you that she was in good health until early this morning when she developed a nonproductive cough and progressively worsening respiratory distress. She has no reported allergies or other medical problems and has not had anything to eat for the past 4 hours.

Physical examination reveals that this 3-year-old girl weighs approximately 35 pounds. She is agitated, diaphoretic, and in serious respiratory distress. Vital signs taken shortly after arrival are BP 110/80, pulse 140, and respiration 34. The conjunctiva, lips, and nail beds all appear dusky. Poor skin turgor is noted, the eyes appear sunken, and the mucous membranes are dry. The oropharynx is clear of foreign debris, vomitus, and secretions. Respiratory excursion is symmetrical and the thorax is without obvious deformity. On auscultation, breath sounds are diminished bilaterally, with only minimal expiratory wheezes appreciated. Heart sounds are S_1S_2 although distant. Abdominal examination is unremarkable. Neurologically, the patient is agitated, but alert and responsive to her surroundings. The remainder of the examination is noncontributory.

You initiate treatment, begin cardiac monitoring (Figure 25–1), and contact medical control. Although you undertake aggressive treatment and administer appropriate medications, your patient continues to show serious respiratory difficulty with only minimal signs of clinical improvement.

Questions

Read each question carefully, keeping in mind the context of the case under discussion. Select the best answer from the choices presented.

1. Normal weight for a patient such as yours is approximately
   A. 20 lbs

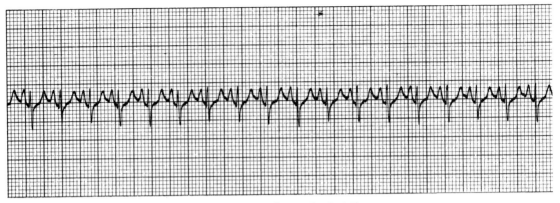

FIGURE 25-1. Lead II EKG recorded shortly after arrival at the scene.

B. 35 lbs
C. 50 lbs
D. 65 lbs

2. Your patient's vital signs are outside the normal range with respect to
   1. Systolic blood pressure
   2. Pulse rate
   3. Diastolic blood pressure
   4. Respiratory rate

   A. 1, 2, and 3 are correct
   B. 1 and 3 are correct
   C. 2 and 4 are correct
   D. Only 4 is correct
   E. All of the above are correct

3. Signs of dehydration in the pediatric patient include
   1. Sunken appearance of the eyes
   2. Dry mucous membranes
   3. Poor skin turgor
   4. Decreased urine flow

   A. 1, 2, and 3 are correct
   B. 1 and 3 are correct
   C. 2 and 4 are correct
   D. Only 4 is correct
   E. All of the above are correct

4. Your patient's EKG (Figure 25-1) is best classified as
   A. Sinus tachycardia
   B. Atrial fibrillation
   C. Normal sinus rhythm
   D. Second degree AV block, Mobitz type II

5. The most likely diagnosis in this case is
   A. Asthma
   B. Foreign body obstruction
   C. Acute bacterial epiglottitis
   D. Emphysema

6. Medical management of your patient's problem might include all the following except
   A. Administering supplemental humidified oxygen
   B. Establishing an intravenous line with D5/0.25 normal saline
   C. Administering epinephrine by subcutaneous injection
   D. Administering morphine sulfate, 10 mg, IV push

7. Complications that may develop in your patient include
   1. Hypoxemia
   2. Dehydration
   3. Hypercarbia
   4. Acidosis

   A. 1, 2, and 3 are correct
   B. 1 and 3 are correct
   C. 2 and 4 are correct
   D. Only 4 is correct
   E. All of the above are correct

8. Medications or other substances that may be valuable in treating your patient include
   1. Epinephrine
   2. Aminophylline
   3. Corticosteroids
   4. Oxygen

   A. 1, 2, and 3 are correct
   B. 1 and 3 are correct
   C. 2 and 4 are correct
   D. Only 4 is correct
   E. All of the above are correct

9. Which of the following combinations reflect(s) correct drug dosages and modes of administration?
   1. Epinephrine 1:1,000, 1 mg/kg subcutaneously
   2. Hydrocortisone, 5 mg/kg IV
   3. Isoetharine, 5 ml in 1 ml of saline via nebulization
   4. Aminophylline, 4 mg/kg diluted in D5/W, IV, over 15 minutes

   A. 1, 2, and 3 are correct
   B. 1 and 3 are correct
   C. 2 and 4 are correct

D. Only 4 is correct
E. All of the above are correct

10. The term *status asthmaticus* refers to
    A. A patient who experiences recurrent bouts of asthma
    B. Asthma that has its onset in early childhood
    C. An asthmatic attack of greater than 1 hour duration
    D. A severe asthmatic attack that does not respond to standard medications

Discussion

This patient presents with an acute onset of respiratory distress that is both severe and progressive. Although there are several important causes of respiratory distress in the pediatric patient, in this case the clinical history and physical examination strongly support a diagnosis of a severe asthma attack (see "Common Causes of Respiratory Distress in Pediatric Patients").

Common Causes of Respiratory Distress in Pediatric Patients

Asthma

Characterized by a generalized hyperreactivity of the airways resulting in episodic reversible airways obstruction. Onset frequently before age 10; clinical features of dyspnea, cough, and wheezing.

Bronchiolitis

An infectious process of viral etiology resulting in inflammation of the bronchioles. Most common in children under 2 years of age; clinical features of dyspnea and generalized wheezing.

Croup

An infectious process of viral etiology; goes also by the name of laryngotracheobronchitis. Most common in children between 6 months and 4 years of age. Clinical features include dyspnea, stridor ("seal bark"), and hoarseness.

Epiglottitis

An infectious process of bacterial etiology resulting in severe inflammation of the epiglottis and surrounding tissues. Most common in children over age 4. Clinical features include dyspnea, pain on swallowing, drooling, and marked respiratory distress.

Airway Obstruction

Due to blockage of the airway by a foreign object (marble, peanut, toy). Clinical features include dyspnea, stridor, and loss of consciousness if obstruction is complete.

Asthma can be operationally defined as a clinical syndrome characterized by episodes of reversible airway obstruction. Although there is no universally accepted classification of the various forms of asthma, a working classification that is helpful in diagnosing and treating this condition is based on the stimulus that triggers the attack (Figure 25-2). Asthma affects persons of all ages but occurs most frequently in children. Estimates indicate that up to 10% of children in the United States suffer from this clinical entity; over half of all cases have their onset before the age of 10.

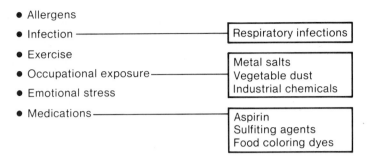

FIGURE 25-2. Factors known to precipitate asthma attacks.

Asthma is characterized by overall increased responsiveness of the tracheobronchial tree to a variety of stimuli. The stimulus that triggers an attack varies from one person to another; stress, exercise, infection, allergens, and other agents can all be potent triggers of asthma in susceptible individuals. Pathophysiologically, an asthma attack results from the combination of constriction of the bronchial smooth muscle, edema and inflammation of the airways, and plugging of the airways with mucous and other debris. The result is *obstruction* of the airways, which produces increased resistance to airflow. This obstructive process is reflected in altered results of pulmonary function tests. Findings include reduced forced vital capacity (FVC), reduced forced expiratory volume in 1 second (FEV_1), and reduced peak expiratory flow rate (PEFR).

With obstruction and increased resistance to flow come the classic clinical features of asthma: cough, wheezing, and dyspnea. In the early phase of an attack the uneven distribution of air (ventilation) and blood flow (perfusion) to the lungs (ventilation-perfusion mismatch) often produces hypoxemia. The patient normally compensates for hypoxemia, pulmonary irritation, and agitation by increasing his respiratory rate and hyperventilating. This tends to "blow off CO_2" and produce a respiratory alkalosis. Blood gas findings during the early stages of an asthma attack classically reveal hypoxemia, hypocapnia, and respiratory alkalosis. As the attack becomes more severe, bronchoconstriction increases, making spontaneous ventilation more difficult. The work of breathing becomes increasingly difficult and the patient may begin to tire. During the late stages of a severe attack, hypoxemia continues, CO_2 retention develops, leading to hypercapnia, and an acidotic state results.

The patient will often complain of severe shortness of breath and pronounced expiratory difficulty. Tachycardia, diaphoresis, and tachypnea are often evident. The patient may appear extremely agitated. Use of accessory muscles to aid in respiration, and other classic signs of respiratory distress, are common. Because of impaired expiration and air trapping, the lungs become hyperinflated, giving the chest an increased anterior-posterior diameter. Percussion will often reveal a hyperresonant note. Auscultation of the lungs may reveal any one of a number of findings, depending on the severity of the attack; generalized wheezing with a significantly prolonged expiratory phase may be seen in some cases, while in others, such as this one, diminished breath sounds are present, with almost no audible wheezes.

Basic life support treatment of your patient should be aimed at ensuring adequate cardiopulmonary function. Administer humidified oxygen to help alleviate hypoxemia. Use a nasal cannula instead of a face mask if necessary (many patients with asthma will not tolerate having a mask strapped over their face). Monitor vital signs with particular attention to the respiratory pattern and blood pressure. Remove any restrictive clothing and encourage the patient to assume the position of greatest comfort.

Advanced life support measures entail constant cardiac monitoring, establishing an intravenous (IV) line, and administering the appropriate medications. Electrocardiogram monitoring is important since hypoxemia and some of the medications used in treating asthma may result in a variety of cardiac arrhythmias. This patient's EKG tracing (Figure 25-1) demonstrates a tachyarrhythmia at a rate of approximately 188 complexes per minute. The presence of P waves defines the rhythm as being of sinus origin, and the constant relationship of atrial P waves to ventricular QRS complexes allows an interpretation of sinus tachycardia. For this patient, however, treatment should focus on the underlying problems rather than the arrhythmia.

Establishing an IV line is important for two reasons. First, it provides a rapid means of administering medications. Second, it allows for fluid replacement. Many patients with asthma show clinical signs of dehydration, so fluid replacement therapy is an important part of treatment. The combined findings in this patient of dry mucous membranes, a sunken appearance of the eyes, and poor skin turgor suggest moderate dehydration. Fluid replacement should be initiated using either D5/W or D5/0.25 normal saline at a rate of 5 to 15 ml/kg/hr.

Medications that may be useful in the management of acute asthma include epinephrine, aminophylline, and corticosteroids. Epinephrine has classically been the first line drug of choice for field treatment of severe asthma. Epinephrine, a β-adrenergic agent, acts to dilate the bronchial smooth musculature by activating β_2-adrenergic receptors. Its clinical effects appear within several minutes after subcutaneous administration, peak in about 20 minutes, and continue for up to 2 hours. Side-effects resulting from stimulation of both α- and β-receptors include:

- Agitation
- Tremor
- Tachycardia
- Pallor
- Palpitations
- Cardiac arrhythmias

In the pediatric patient epinephrine is normally administered subcutaneously as a dose of 0.01 ml/kg, using a 1:1,000 concentration. A second dose may be repeated in 20 minutes if required. Because other medications may interact with or potentiate the effects of epinephrine, it is important to be aware of any and all medicines the patient may take.

Aminophylline is a bronchodilator that belongs to a class of agents known as the methylxanthines. Although their exact mechanism of action is unclear, aminophylline and related agents act in a variety of ways to decrease bronchoconstriction and open the airways. Because there is a narrow margin between the necessary therapeutic dose and one that may cause a toxic reaction, it is extremely important to administer this medication carefully and to watch for signs of toxicity. Correct administration of aminophylline in the pediatric patient who has not recently had aminophylline or related agents calls for 2 to 4 mg/kg, diluted in normal saline and administered intravenously over not less than 15 to 20 minutes.

Corticosteroids, although more effective in preventing attacks and in treating chronic asthma, are also frequently employed in cases of status asthmaticus. Hydrocortisone is commonly administered intravenously as a 5 mg/kg dose.

Following initial treatment, continue frequent monitoring of your patient's vital signs, clinical status, and cardiac rhythm during transport to the hospital.

Field Diagnosis

- Acute respiratory distress
- Status asthmaticus

Hospital Diagnosis

- Status asthmaticus
- Dehydration

Patient Follow-Up

Following transport to the emergency room, your patient continued to demonstrate increasing respiratory distress. Arterial blood gases measured in the hospital revealed a respiratory acidosis with marked hypoxemia. Despite aggressive treatment with sympathomimetic agents, steroids, and inhalational bronchodilators, your patient continued to demonstrate increasing hypercapnia and hypoxemia. A decision was made to intubate the patient and provide ventilatory support. After 6 days in the pediatric intensive care unit, your patient was discharged from the hospital on medication.

Answers

1. B

   Behrman RE, Vaughan VC III, Nelson WC: Textbook of Pediatrics, 12th ed, p. 27. Philadelphia, WB Saunders, 1983

2. C

   Behrman RE, Vaughan VC III, Nelson WC: Textbook of Pediatrics, 12th ed, pp 1100–1102. Philadelphia, WB Saunders, 1983
   Caroline NL: Emergency Care in the Streets, 3rd ed, p 519. Boston, Little, Brown & Co, 1987

   Grant HD, Murray RH Jr, Bergeron JD: Emergency Care, 4th ed, p 376. Englewood Cliffs, NJ, Prentice-Hall, 1986

3. E

   Behrman RE, Vaughan VC III, Nelson WC: Textbook of Pediatrics, 12th ed, p 234. Philadelphia, WB Saunders, 1983
   Caroline NL: Emergency Care in the Streets, 3rd ed, p 511. Boston, Little, Brown & Co, 1987

4. A

Huff J, Doernbach DP, White RD: ECG Workout: Exercises in Arrhythmia Interpretation, pp 13, 213 (strip 1.25). Philadelphia, JB Lippincott, 1985

5. A

Caroline NL: Emergency Care in the Streets, 3rd ed, pp 510-512. Boston, Little, Brown & Co, 1987

Grant HD, Murray RH Jr, Bergeron JD: Emergency Care, 4th ed, pp 382-383. Englewood Cliffs, NJ, Prentice-Hall, 1986

Behrman RE, Vaughan VC III, Nelson WC: Textbook of Pediatrics, 12th ed, pp 541-542. Philadelphia, WB Saunders, 1983

6. D

Caroline NL: Emergency Care in the Streets, 3rd ed, pp 148, 510-511. Boston, Little, Brown & Co, 1987

7. E

Caroline NL: Emergency Care in the Streets, 3rd ed, p 510. Boston, Little, Brown & Co, 1987

Behrman RE, Vaughan VC III, Nelson WC: Textbook of Pediatrics, 12th ed, pp 544-545. Philadelphia, WB Saunders, 1983

8. E

Behrman RE, Vaughan VC III, Nelson WC: Textbook of Pediatrics, 12th ed, pp 544-545. Philadelphia, WB Saunders, 1983

Caroline NL: Emergency Care in the Streets, 3rd ed, pp 511-512. Boston, Little, Brown & Co, 1987

9. C

Caroline NL: Emergency Care in the Streets, 3rd ed, p 512. Boston, Little, Brown & Co, 1987

Behrman RE, Vaughan VC III, Nelson WC: Textbook of Pediatrics, 12th ed, pp 544-545. Philadelphia, WB Saunders, 1983

10. D

Behrman RE, Vaughan VC III, Nelson WC: Textbook of Pediatrics, 12th ed, p 544. Philadelphia, WB Saunders, 1983

Caroline NL: Emergency Care in the Streets, 3rd ed, p 510. Boston, Little, Brown & Co, 1987

Selected Reading

Downie RL: Obstructive airway disease. In Taliaferro EH: Respiratory Emergencies. Top Emerg Med 8:13, 1987

Miech RP, Stein M: Methylxanthines. In Ziment I, Popa V (eds): Respiratory Pharmacology. Clin Chest Med 7:331, 1986

Popa V: Beta-Adrenergic Drugs. In Ziment I, Popa V (eds): Respiratory Pharmacology. Clin Chest Med 7:313, 1986

Stibolt TB Jr: Asthma In Bone RC (ed): Medical Emergencies I. Med Clin North Am 70:909, 1986

Ziment I: Steroids. In Ziment I, Popa V (eds): Respiratory Pharmacology. Clin Chest Med 7:341, 1986

OBSTETRIC– GYNECOLOGIC EMERGENCIES

26

Abdominal Pain, Weakness, and Hypotension in a Teenage Woman

Your ambulance is called for a woman with severe abdominal pain. Upon arrival, you discover your patient lying in bed, agitated, and sweating. Her family is present and very concerned. The parents tell you that their daughter awoke this morning with severe abdominal pain, started to sweat profusely, and nearly passed out while she was walking to the bathroom. After helping her back to bed, they called EMS. They state that she is rarely sick and has never been this ill. As your partner continues talking with the parents, you begin directly questioning the patient and initiate your physical examination.

The patient is an 18-year-old woman who appears pale, extremely diaphoretic, and in obvious pain. She tells you that her pain started approximately 3 hours ago, is most intense in the lower right quadrant, and is minimally radiating. She describes the pain as "sharp, intense, and stabbing." It is associated with lightheadedness, nausea, and sweating, and is not relieved by simple self-administered analgesics. Although she is not eager to answer this question, your patient reports that she is not sexually active and does not use birth control. Her menstrual cycles are normally regular, but her last menstrual period was 8 weeks ago.

Medical history includes a childhood heart murmur and a recent sore throat. Medications are limited to recently-prescribed penicillin, 250 mg po qid. She has no allergies and no significant alcohol or tobacco history.

Upon examination, her initial vital signs reveal BP (left arm, supine) 90/60, pulse 120 and regular, respiration 26 and regular, and temperature cool to touch. Vital signs repeated with the patient in a sitting position show BP 80 by palpation, pulse 140 regular and thready, respiration 26 and regular, and temperature cool to touch. Head and neck are remarkable for a pharyngeal exudate and very pale conjunctiva. Heart and lung examination do not produce abnormal findings. The abdomen appears normal in shape and contour and is nondistended. No surgical scars are noted either anteriorly or posteriorly. Bowel sounds are absent in all four quadrants despite continued auscultation. Marked guarding is noted during palpation and is most prominent on the right side. No masses are felt. Significant rebound tenderness is discovered in all abdominal quadrants but is more severe on the right. Extremities show no signs of clubbing, cyanosis, or edema, although capillary refill is delayed. Your patient is neurologically intact with pupils round, equal, and reactive to light.

Obstetric–Gynecologic Emergencies

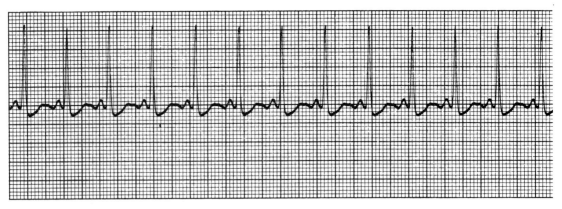

FIGURE 26-1. Lead II EKG recorded shortly after arrival at the scene.

You institute field treatment, record your patient's cardiac rhythm (Figure 26-1), and contact medical control. Transport begins and treatment continues, while monitoring of vital signs and cardiac rhythm is maintained. Vital signs repeated 5 minutes into transport are BP (left arm, supine) 88/58, pulse 110 regular and weak, and respiration 24 and regular. Your receiving hospital is notified of your imminent arrival and transport continues.

Upon arrival in the emergency room, your patient is alert, with a blood pressure of 90/60 and a pulse of 110. Her hematocrit is 28. A transfusion of packed red blood cells (RBCs) is initiated while the operating room is placed on standby.

Questions

Read each question carefully, keeping in mind the context of the case under discussion. Select the best answer from the choices presented.

1. Which of the following common medical suffixes is *not* paired with its correct meaning?
   A. *-itis*   .... inflammation of
   B. *-algia*   .... pain in
   C. *-megaly* .... weakness
   D. *-oma*   .... tumor of

2. Which of the following structures is not considered part of the female reproductive system?
   A. Ovaries
   B. Uterus
   C. Prostate gland
   D. Cervix

3. Your patient's presenting problem is best summarized by the term

A. Acute abdomen
B. Myocardial ischemia
C. Cor pulmonale
D. Rapid buildup of ascites

4. Common causes of severe abdominal pain include
   1. Cholecystitis
   2. Ectopic pregnancy
   3. Appendicitis
   4. Dissecting abdominal aortic aneurysm

   A. 1, 2, and 3 are correct
   B. 1 and 3 are correct
   C. 2 and 4 are correct
   D. Only 4 is correct
   E. All are correct

5. Which of the following conditions characteristically begins with periumbilical pain and anorexia?
   A. Cholecystitis
   B. Acute appendicitis
   C. Pelvic inflammatory disease
   D. Ectopic pregnancy

6. Which of the following statements about acute appendicitis is *incorrect*?
   A. Most patients demonstrate anorexia, right lower quadrant abdominal pain, and vomiting
   B. The early pain is often located periumbilically and later radiates to the right lower abdominal quadrant
   C. The patient often has an associated fever
   D. Initial treatment calls for high-dose antibiotic therapy; surgery is necessary only if antibiotics are ineffective

7. Which of the following clinical findings may help support a diagnosis of dissecting aortic aneurysm?
   A. Paroxysmal atrial tachycardia
   B. Upper extremity inequality in blood pressure or pulse
   C. Periods of Cheyne-Stokes respiration
   D. Lower extremity pedal edema

8. Which of the following sets of clues is most helpful in determining the specific etiology of your patient's condition?
   A. Female sex, age of 18, date of last menstrual period
   B. Associated nausea, hypotension, diaphoresis
   C. Female sex, age of 18, recent use of penicillin
   D. History of a heart murmur, right-sided abdominal pain, age of 18

9. In a young woman with abdominal pain the report of a missed menstrual period most suggests
    A. Cholecystitis
    B. Perforated ulcer
    C. Ectopic pregnancy
    D. Gonorrhea

10. The absence of bowel sounds in this patient is
    A. Probably normal and of no significance
    B. Probably abnormal and suggests peritonitis
    C. Normal and expected in a patient taking penicillin
    D. Abnormal and found in the vast majority of patients with hypotension

11. The best working field diagnosis in this case is
    A. Ruptured ectopic pregnancy
    B. Pelvic inflammatory disease
    C. Acute appendicitis
    D. Acute cholecystitis
    E. Ruptured abdominal aortic aneurysm

12. Basic life support treatment of your patient should include
    1. Administering supplemental oxygen
    2. Delaying transport and preparing the patient for childbirth
    3. Placing patient in Trendelenburg position
    4. Applying venous constricting bands

    A. 1, 2, and 3 are correct
    B. 1 and 3 are correct
    C. 2 and 4 are correct
    D. Only 4 is correct
    E. All are correct

13. Which of the following oxygen delivery systems will deliver a 35% to 60% enriched oxygen mixture?
    A. Nasal cannula at 2 to 4 1/min
    B. Non-rebreathing mask at 10 to 12 1/min
    C. Partial rebreathing mask at 6 to 10 1/min
    D. Non-rebreathing mask at 2 to 4 1/min

14. The most immediate problem requiring correction in your patient is
    A. Hypovolemia
    B. Sepsis
    C. Hypoxia
    D. Cardiac arrhythmia

15. Advanced life support treatment of your patient should include
    1. Establishment of peripheral intravenous lines

2. Cardiac monitoring
3. Application of MAST
4. Immediate intubation

A. 1, 2, and 3 are correct
B. 1 and 3 are correct
C. 2 and 4 are correct
D. Only 4 is correct
E. All are correct

16. Which of the following medications are indicated in the treatment of your patient?
    1. Naloxone, 0.4 mg, slow IV push
    2. Morphine sulfate, 2 mg, slow IV push
    3. Thiamine, 50 mg, IV push
    4. Intravenous fluids

    A. 1, 2, and 3 are correct
    B. 1 and 3 are correct
    C. 2 and 4 are correct
    D. Only 4 is correct
    E. All are correct

17. Which of the following intravenous set-ups is most desirable for your patient?
    A. External jugular vein cannulation with a 20-gauge needle
    B. Two 22-gauge peripheral intravenous anticubital lines
    C. Internal jugular vein cannulation with an 18-gauge needle
    D. Two 16-gauge peripheral intravenous lines

18. The fluid of choice for this patient would be
    A. Lactated Ringer's
    B. D5/W
    C. 0.45% normal saline in dextrose
    D. 10% dextrose

19. Complications that may result from intravenous therapy include
    1. Pyrogenic reactions
    2. Infiltration
    3. Air embolism
    4. Infection

    A. 1, 2, and 3 are correct
    B. 1 and 3 are correct
    C. 2 and 4 are correct
    D. Only 4 is correct
    E. All are correct

20. Your patient's initial cardiac rhythm (Figure 26-1) is abnormal with respect to

A. Rate
B. Rhythm
C. Morphology of the complexes
D. Interval durations

21. The physiological cause of your patient's cardiac arrhythmia is most likely
    A. Recent use of penicillin
    B. A compensatory response to hypovolemia
    C. Peritoneal inflammation
    D. A vagal response to pain

22. Your patient's initial cardiac rhythm (Figure 26-1) is best classified as
    A. Normal sinus rhythm
    B. Second degree AV block
    C. Atrial fibrillation
    D. Sinus tachycardia

23. Following initial treatment of your patient, vital signs are repeated 5 minutes into transport and show BP 88/58, pulse 110 regular and weak, and respiration 24 and regular. Your next course of action should be
    A. Establish a dopamine infusion at 5 ug/kg/min
    B. Perform synchronized DC cardioversion at 50 Joules
    C. Monitor vital signs and continue fluid replacement
    D. Establish an isoproterenol infusion at 2 ug/min

24. An *ectopic pregnancy* is best defined as
    A. Premature implantation of an embryo or fetus in the uterus
    B. Implantation of an embryo or fetus anywhere outside the uterus
    C. Intrauterine death of an embryo or fetus
    D. Premature rupture of the fetal membranes

25. Which of the following in-hospital procedures is useful in evaluating the patient with a suspected ruptured ectopic pregnancy?
    A. Abdominal CT scan
    B. Amniocentesis
    C. Lumbar puncture
    D. Culdocentesis

Discussion

Ectopic pregnancy is a potentially life-threatening situation that must always be seriously considered in any female patient of reproductive age who complains of abdominal pain (see "Important Clinical Features of Ectopic Pregnancy"). *Ectopic pregnancy* refers to a pregnancy in which the embryo or fetus implants and develops outside of the uterus. Implantation may occur in one of several sites, including the cervix, fallopian tube, ovary, or abdominal cavity. Because the most

Important Clinical Features of Ectopic Pregnancy

Definition

Implantation of the fertilized ovum outside of the uterine cavity.

Site of Implantation

Frequency	Location
Most common ↓	Fallopian tube
	• Ampullar region
	• Isthmic region
	Ovarian
	Abdominal
Least common	Cervical

Epidemiology

Ectopic pregnancy has a frequency of approximately 1 in every 100–200 births. Approximately 1 in 20 cases results in death secondary to hemorrhage.

Risk Factors

Pelvic inflammatory disease, IUD, previous pelvic surgery, tubal ligation

Clinical Manifestations

HISTORY	SIGNS AND SYMPTOMS*
Lower abdominal pain	Severe lower abdominal pain
Abnormal LMP	Weakness, dizziness, syncope
Risk factor (see above)	Abdominal tenderness and guarding
Spotty vaginal bleeding	Signs of hypovolemic shock
	• Tachycardia
	• Pallor
	• Hypotension
	• Diaphoresis

*Seen with rupture

common site of implantation is within the narrow confines of the fallopian tube, a frequent complication in ectopic pregnancy is rupture of the tube with massive hemorrhage. This complication occurs most often during the first 8 to 10 weeks of pregnancy, when the growth of the fetus causes excessive stretching of the narrow lumen of the fallopian tube. The resulting rupture often causes extensive internal hemorrhage, major blood loss, and frank hemorrhagic shock.

Recognizing an ectopic pregnancy centers around both careful questioning of the patient and a good physical examination. In any female patient complaining of abdominal pain, certain key questions must be raised. First, is the patient sexually active and, if so, how recently? Interpret the patient's response to this question carefully, because it is not uncommon for patients to either deny or exaggerate their sexual activity. It is often advisable, especially when dealing with a young patient in a family setting, to question her discreetly and apart from her parents. Second, does the patient use contraceptives? If so, remember that certain contraceptive devices, such as the intrauterine device (IUD), may predispose the patient to pelvic inflammatory disease with consequent abscess formation and perforation. Third, a careful gynecologic history may reveal factors that are known to predispose to ectopic pregnancy, such as a prior ectopic pregnancy or constant and recurrent pelvic inflammatory disease. Finally, the date of the last menstrual period (LMP) is of great importance. Although there are many causes of a late or missed menstrual period, taken in the proper setting, such a finding must always raise the possibility of an ectopic pregnancy.

Physical findings associated with a ruptured ectopic pregnancy vary, but certain signs are characteristic. Abdominal pain will often be of sudden onset, hypogastric in location, and either unilateral or bilateral. The rupture of the fallopian tube results in peritonitis with guarding, tenderness, rebound, and often frank abdominal rigidity. Additionally, the associated decreased gut motility may produce the finding of absent or decreased bowel sounds, as in this patient. Hypovolemia resulting from loss of blood into the peritoneal cavity may produce pronounced signs, including hypotension, orthostatic changes, tachycardia, syncope, nausea, and vomiting.

Although an acute abdomen with serious hypotension may have several etiologies, its presentation in a young, probably sexually active woman who reports a missed menstrual period, as in this case, strongly suggests a ruptured ectopic pregnancy. Your field diagnosis is thus hemorrhagic shock secondary to a probable ruptured ectopic pregnancy. The primary goal of treatment is correcting the hypovolemia and associated shock state. Because your patient is conscious and breathing spontaneously, she is not a candidate for either assisted ventilation or intubation; supplemental oxygen administration is satisfactory. Her cardiac rhythm shows an appropriate sinus tachycardia, probably compensatory in nature, and without ectopy. Specific treatment of the cardiac arrhythmia is not necessary. Aggressive measures to correct the underlying hypovolemia are necessary, however, and should include applying military antishock trousers (MAST) and establishing an intravenous (IV) route. In cases such as this where there has been massive blood loss, it is preferable to establish at least two large-bore (14- or 16-gauge catheters) peripheral IV lines, using an administration set designed for rapid administration of fluids ("macro drip"). Volume replacement should involve a fluid designed to expand intravascular volume. In the field this is best accomplished by using either a colloid such as human plasma protein fraction (Plasmanate), or a crystalloid solution such as lactated Ringer's or normal saline (the two most commonly employed). Additional hemodynamic support may be gained by applying MAST, which may act both to increase blood pressure and to limit further internal bleeding.

Following these measures, your patient shows signs of hemodynamic stabilization. Hence the use of vasopressor agents such as dopamine or norepinephrine should be deferred. Instead, continue fluid replacement and constantly monitor vital signs and cardiac rhythm. Rapid transport to a nearby medical facility is mandatory so that further evaluation and definitive treatment can be provided.

> **Field Diagnosis**
> - Hypovolemic shock
> - Acute abdomen
>
> **Hospital Diagnosis**
> - Ectopic pregnancy with rupture

Patient Follow-Up

The patient's condition was evaluated by the obstetrical team, who considered a culdocentesis (Figure 26–2) but, due to her unstable condition, elected instead to transport her to the operating room for an emergency exploratory laparotomy. Exploration revealed an ectopic pregnancy in the ampulla of the right fallopian tube. In addition, one liter of blood was removed from the peritoneal cavity. The patient tolerated surgery well and was discharged from the hospital after an uneventful postoperative course.

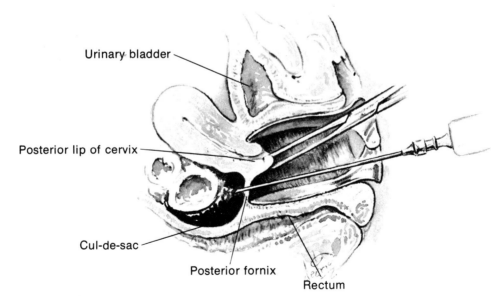

FIGURE 26–2. Cul-de-sac aspiration. The posterior fornix is infiltrated with local anesthetic agent. A 4-inch needle attached to a syringe is inserted into the cul-de-sac parallel with the spine. If nonclotting blood is recovered, the tap is positive. (Cosgriff JH Jr, Anderson DL: The Practice of Emergency Care, 2nd ed, p 460. Philadelphia, JB Lippincott, 1984)

Answers

1. **C**
   Caroline NL: Emergency Care in the Streets, 3rd ed, p 15. Boston, Little, Brown & Co, 1987

2. **C**
   Caroline NL: Emergency Care in the Streets, 3rd ed, p 37. Boston, Little, Brown & Co, 1987

3. **A**
   Caroline NL: Emergency Care in the Streets, 3rd ed, pp 456–459. Boston, Little, Brown & Co, 1987

4. **E**
   Caroline NL: Emergency Care in the Streets, 3rd ed, pp 456–459. Boston, Little, Brown & Co, 1987
   Caroline NL: Emergency Medical Treatment: A Text for EMT-As and EMT-Intermediates, 2nd ed, pp 403–407. Boston, Little, Brown & Co, 1987

5. **B**
   Caroline NL: Emergency Medical Treatment: A Text for EMT-As and EMT-Intermediates, 2nd ed, pp 403–405. Boston, Little, Brown & Co, 1987
   Krome RL: Acute appendicitis. In Tintinalli JE, Rothstein RJ, Krome RL (eds): Emergency Medicine: A Comprehensive Study Guide. New York, McGraw-Hill, 1985

6. **D**
   Krome RL: Acute appendicitis. In Tintinalli JE, Rothstein RJ, Krome RL (eds): Emergency Medicine: A Comprehensive Study Guide. New York, McGraw-Hill, 1985

7. **B**
   Caroline NL: Emergency Care in the Streets, 3rd ed, p 459. Boston, Little, Brown & Co, 1987
   Feldman AJ: Thoracic and abdominal aortic aneurysms. In Tintinalli JE, Rothstein RJ, Krome RL (eds): Emergency Medicine: A Comprehensive Study Guide. New York, McGraw-Hill, 1985
   Szilagyi DE: Clinical diagnosis of intact and ruptured abdominal aneurysms. In Bergan JJ, Yao JST (eds): Aneurysms: Diagnosis and Treatment. New York, Grune & Stratton, 1982

8. **A**
   Caroline NL: Emergency Care in the Streets, 3rd ed, pp 482–484. Boston, Little, Brown & Co, 1987
   Hockberger RS: Obstetric emergencies. In Tintinalli JE, Rothstein RJ, Krome RL (eds): Emergency Medicine: A Comprehensive Study Guide. New York, McGraw-Hill, 1985

9. **C**
   Caroline NL: Emergency Care in the Streets, 3rd ed, pp 482–484. Boston, Little, Brown & Co, 1987
   Hockberger RS: Obstetric emergencies. In Tintinalli JE, Rothstein RJ, Krome RL (eds): Emergency Medicine: A Comprehensive Study Guide. New York, McGraw-Hill, 1985

10. **B**
    Caroline NL: Emergency Care in the Streets, 3rd ed, pp 50–51, 458–459. Boston, Little, Brown & Co, 1987

11. **A**
    Caroline NL: Emergency Care in the Streets, 3rd ed, pp 482–484. Boston, Little, Brown & Co, 1987
    Hockberger RS: Obstetric emergencies. In Tintinalli JE, Rothstein RJ, Krome RL (eds): Emergency Medicine: A Comprehensive Study Guide. New York, McGraw-Hill, 1985
    Iffy L: Ectopic pregnancy. In Edlich RF, Spyker DA, Haury BB (eds): Current Emergency Therapy, 3rd ed. Rockville, MD, Aspen, 1986

12. **B**
    Caroline NL: Emergency Care in the Streets, 3rd ed, pp 482–483. Boston, Little, Brown & Co, 1987

13. **C**
    Caroline NL: Emergency Care in the Streets, 3rd ed, pp 216–219. Boston, Little, Brown & Co, 1987

14. **A**
    Caroline NL: Emergency Care in the Streets, 3rd ed, pp 482–484. Boston, Little, Brown & Co, 1987

15. **A**
    Caroline NL: Emergency Care in the Streets, 3rd ed, pp 482–484. Boston, Little, Brown & Co, 1987
    Hockberger RS: Obstetric emergencies. In Tintinalli JE, Rothstein RJ, Krome RL (eds): Emergency Medicine: A Comprehensive Study Guide. New York, McGraw-Hill, 1985

Iffy L: Ectopic pregnancy. In Edlich RF, Spyker DA, Haury BB (eds): Current Emergency Therapy, 3rd ed. Rockville, MD, Aspen, 1986

16. D

Caroline NL: Emergency Care in the Streets, 3rd ed, pp 482–484. Boston, Little, Brown & Co, 1987

Hockberger RS: Obstetric emergencies. In Tintinalli JE, Rothstein RJ, Krome RL (eds): Emergency Medicine: A Comprehensive Study Guide. New York, McGraw-Hill, 1985

Iffy L: Ectopic pregnancy. In Edlich RF, Spyker DA, Haury BB (eds): Current Emergency Therapy, 3rd ed. Rockville, MD, Aspen, 1986

17. D

Caroline NL: Emergency Care in the Streets, 3rd ed, p 483. Boston, Little, Brown & Co, 1987

18. A

Caroline NL: Emergency Care in the Streets, 3rd ed, p 483. Boston, Little, Brown & Co, 1987

19. E

Caroline NL: Emergency Care in the Streets, 3rd ed, pp 87–88. Boston, Little, Brown & Co, 1987

20. A

Huff J, Doernbach DP, White RD: ECG Workout: Exercises in Arrhythmia Interpretation, p 8 (strip 1.10). Philadelphia, JB Lippincott, 1985

21. B

Caroline NL: Emergency Care in the Streets, 3rd ed, p 78–83. Boston, Little, Brown & Co, 1987

22. D

Huff J, Doernbach DP, White RD: ECG Workout: Exercises in Arrhythmia Interpretation, p 8 (strip 1.10). Philadelphia, JB Lippincott, 1985

23. C

Caroline NL: Emergency Care in the Streets, 3rd ed, pp 78–83. Boston, Little, Brown & Co, 1987

24. B

Caroline NL: Emergency Care in the Streets, 3rd ed, pp 482–483. Boston, Little, Brown & Co, 1987

25. D

Hockberger RS: Obstetric emergencies. In Tintinalli JE, Rothstein RJ, Krome RL (eds): Emergency Medicine: A Comprehensive Study Guide. New York, McGraw-Hill, 1985

Iffy L: Ectopic pregnancy. In Edlich RF, Spyker DA, Haury BB (eds): Current Emergency Therapy, 3rd ed. Rockville, MD, Aspen, 1986

Selected Reading

Brenner PF et al: Ectopic pregnancy: A study of 300 consecutive surgically treated cases. JAMA 243:673, 1980

Hammond CB: Gynecology: Uterus, ovaries, and vagina. In Sabiston DC Jr (ed): Textbook of Surgery, 13th ed. Philadelphia, WB Saunders, 1986

Hockberger RS: Obstetric emergencies. In Tintinalli JE, Rothstein RJ, Krome RL (eds): Emergency Medicine: A Comprehensive Study Guide. New York, McGraw-Hill, 1985

Iffy L: Ectopic pregnancy. In Edlich RF, Spyker DA, Haury BB (eds): Current Emergency Therapy, 3rd ed. Rockville, MD, Aspen, 1986

McElin TW, Iffy L: Ectopic gestation: Consideration of new and controversial issues relating to pathogenesis and management. In Wynn RM (ed): Obstetrics and Gynecology Annual, Vol 5. New York, Appleton-Century-Crofts, 1976